Respiratory Physiology for the Intensivist

Respiratory Physiology for the Intensivist

...

Robert L. Vender, MD

© 2016 **Robert L. Vender, MD**
All rights reserved.

ISBN-10: **1530352630**
ISBN 13: **9781530352630**
Library of Congress Control Number: **2016907323**
CreateSpace Independent Publishing Platform
North Charleston, South Carolina

Contents

Acknowledgments · vii
Preface ·ix
    General ICU Principles · x
    Terminology/Definitions/Abbreviations · · · · · · · · · · · xii
Introduction ·xxi

Chapter 1   Carbon Dioxide (CO_2) · 1
Chapter 2   Oxygen (O_2) · 8
Chapter 3   Pulmonary Gas Exchange · · · · · · · · · · · · · · · · · · · 15
Chapter 4   Hypercapnia · 21
Chapter 5   Hypoxemia · 26
Chapter 6   The Upper Airway · 32
Chapter 7   Mechanics · 39
    Transpulmonary Pressure and Static
    Pressure/Volume Relationship · · · · · · · · · · · · · · · · · · 39
    Lung/Chest Wall Compliance and Elastance · · · · · · · · 45
    Airway Resistance and the Dynamic
    Phase of Breathing/Respiration · · · · · · · · · · · · · · · · · 51
    Work of Breathing · 53
Chapter 8   Pulmonary Circulation · 65
Chapter 9   Control of Ventilation and Central Respiratory Drive · · · 74
Chapter 10 Respiratory Muscles · 83
Chapter 11 Abnormalities of the Chest Wall · · · · · · · · · · · · · · · 95
    Abnormal respiratory mechanics in kyphoscoliosis · · · · 96
    Abnormal gas exchange in kyphoscoliosis · · · · · · · · · · · 98

Chapter 12 Pleural Effusion/Pneumothorax/Ascites · · · · · · · · · · · · · · 101
            Pleural Effusion · 101
            Abnormal Gas Exchange in Pleural Effusion · · · · · · · 102
            Abnormal Respiratory Mechanics in
            Pleural Effusion · 102
            Pneumothorax · 104
            Ascites · 105
Chapter 13 Venous-Thromboembolic Disease · · · · · · · · · · · · · · · · · · 110
            Abnormal Gas Exchange in
            Pulmonary Embolism · 111
Chapter 14 Obstructive Airways Diseases · 116
            Chronic Obstructive Pulmonary Disease · · · · · · · · · · 116
            Abnormal Gas Exchange in COPD · · · · · · · · · · · · · · · 119
            Asthma · 123
            Abnormal Respiratory Mechanics in
            Obstructive Airway Disease (Asthma and COPD) · · · 126
Chapter 15 Acute Respiratory Distress Syndrome · · · · · · · · · · · · · · · 142
            Abnormal Gas Exchange in ARDS · · · · · · · · · · · · · · · 144
            Abnormal Respiratory Mechanics in ARDS · · · · · · · · 146
Chapter 16 Severe Community-Acquired Pneumonia · · · · · · · · · · · · 156
            Abnormal Gas Exchange in Acute
            Bacterial Pneumonia · 157
Chapter 17 Blunt Chest Trauma · 160
            Pulmonary Contusion · 160
            Flail Chest · 163
Chapter 18 Extreme/Morbid Obesity · 166
Chapter 19 Cystic Fibrosis · 176
            Abnormal Gas Exchange in Cystic Fibrosis · · · · · · · · · 178
            Abnormal Respiratory Mechanics in
            Cystic Fibrosis · 179

            About the Author · 183

Acknowledgments

• • •

I HUMBLY ACKNOWLEDGE THE FOLLOWING individuals who guided my path—but more importantly, forged who I am: my wife, Lucina; Stephanie; Jonathan; Robert; Benjamin; Henry; my mother, Martha; my father, Louis; Uncle John; Joseph; and Mary Lou.

Preface

• • •

Though I acknowledge significant technological advancements relating to instrumentation, mechanical ventilation, and monitoring devices in the critical-care setting, their application in clinical medicine remains founded in the same physiological principles applied over the past fifty years. Surprisingly, these scientific advancements have resulted in only relatively minor improvements in patient mortality and even less-convincing improvements in morbidity and quality of life. In fact, extensive debate still exists in relation to the overall individual patient and societal benefits of modern acute critical care and has assisted in the rebirth of the specialty of palliative care medicine. Again, surprisingly, the only universally accepted standard of care or guideline generated from this advanced technology relates to a single clinical entity, that being the "lung protection strategy" of mechanical ventilation for patients with acute respiratory distress syndrome (ARDS), originally referred to as the adult respiratory distress syndrome. Nevertheless, there clearly exist unique applications of respiratory physiology theory and practice as applies specifically to the unique population of critically ill patients requiring intensive-care unit (ICU) care, especially as relates to invasive mechanical ventilation. The purpose of this manual is to concisely review key physiological principles to aid in the understanding of recent technological advancements in the ICU setting, obviously with the ultimate goal to improve the clinical outcomes of all patients seeking, electing, or requiring the specialty practice of ICU medicine. These various physiological principles in both health and disease have translated into specific aspects of ventilator management unique to specific disease entities.

This publication contains no original author-generated studies or investigations but draws information from the myriad of dedicated and extremely knowledgeable individuals whose lifelong career goals and accomplishments were in the field of respiratory physiology. I acknowledge the simplistic approach taken in this book and also acknowledge potential errors or inaccuracies in the interpretation of published articles, texts, and reviews. I have made every attempt to provide accurate, concise information, which I am sure I have not fully accomplished. However, the key goal is to bring to life, in the real world and in real time, these physiological principles in the practice of critical-care medicine. Hopefully, this will stimulate each individual reader's enthusiasm to pursue these concepts with much greater depth while neither implicating nor recommending any specific clinical practice patterns or guidelines.

General ICU Principles

1. Many physiological functions are nonlinear but rather hyperbolic or exponential in nature, with the resulting corollary that it takes a large volume or profusion of disease to clinically deteriorate from "good" to "bad" but only minor worsening of that disease to transition from "bad" to "worse."
2. One of the worse diagnoses prognostically in the ICU is "no" diagnosis—that is, an absence of a diagnosis.
3. For each individual ICU patient, there is no such terminology as "normal" physiological variables or parameters but rather what is necessary in the "diseased" state to maintain survivability, noting that many ICU patients will die with "normal" physiological measurements; conversely many ICU patients will survive with "abnormal" physiological mesaurements.

4. Every case of acute respiratory failure is always a combination of an imbalance of requisite work of breathing and the strength and endurance of the respiratory muscles.
5. Despite the simplistic description of the lung functioning as a single uniform/homogeneous unit, it must certainly be acknowledged that each individual airway and each alveolar unit functions as a distinct entity with remarkable heterogeneity both in health and disease, for which regional variability becomes especially aggravated in diseased lungs.
6. Despite the focus on the respiratory system, all organs and all systems are integrally linked in a single overall body homeostasis where each individual component interacts with each other component to affect not only individual systems outcomes but, even more importantly, overall patient morbidity and mortality.
7. The words "static" or "status quo" should not exist in the vocabulary of ICU medicine, given the extreme fluidity of patient physiology and minute-to-minute changes and variations.
8. As critical-care providers, it is also our responsibility to think beyond the patients' immediate care and consider their subsequent outcomes and livelihood for one year, five years, and even ten years after discharge from the ICU and not simply limit our clinical duties to those few days of critical illness, which are a mere fraction of the patients' entire overall lifespan.
9. From a time and temporal perspective, nothing in the ICU terminology stands for "acute," as numerous treatments are for chronic diseases and chronic durations of care, even in an ICU setting.
10. At times in the ICU, some interventions are the patients' "friends" but at other times their "enemies," noting the importance of monitoring for this transition point, such as too much / too long duration sedation, antibiotic administration, or prolonged mechanical ventilation.

11. The hardest patients to extubate are those who cannot tell you that you made a mistake—that is, the population vulnerable because of neurological disease or disordered mentation.
12. Often the mechanism or disease cause that initiates and precipitates acute respiratory failure is not the same mechanism or disease process that maintains or perpetuates the chronic requirement for invasive mechanical ventilation, especially in relation to the development of ICU-acquired weakness and the clinical syndrome of the chronic critically ill.
13. Critical-care providers should be prepared to reset priorities upon overall recovery (mental, physical, functional, and psychological) and not simply survival.

Terminology/Definitions/Abbreviations

A: alveolar

a: arterial

A-aO$_2$ gradient: alveolar-arterial oxygen difference/gradient; calculated as the difference between an ABG determined PaO$_2$ and the alveolar PAO$_2$ with PAO$_2$ defined as equal to (FiO$_2$ × [Patm − PH$_2$O]) − PaCO$_2$/RQ (respiratory quotient), where normal A-aO$_2$ gradient is less than 12

AECOPD: acute exacerbation of chronic obstructive pulmonary disease

ARDS: acute respiratory distress syndrome

ARF: acute respiratory failure

BB: blue bloater; descriptive of COPD patient phenotype presumed dominated by the chronic bronchitis clinical phenotype associated with hypercapnia, hypoxemia, and cor pulmonale

BiPAP: bilevel positive airway pressure; characterized by defined preset levels of inspiratory (IPAP) and expiratory (EPAP) positive-pressure settings

BMI: body mass index (kg/m^2)

CaO$_2$: arterial oxygen content/concentration (usually expressed as mL O$_2$/100 mL blood); in healthy subjects, approximately 20 mL O$_2$/100 mL blood (20 vol %) and calculated as (1.39 mLO$_2$ × Hgb × % saturation) + (0.003 × PaO$_2$)—the latter component representing only approximately 2 percent of entire CaO$_2$

CaCO$_2$: arterial carbon dioxide content/concentration (usually expressed as mL CO$_2$/100 mL blood), which value is dependent upon PaCO$_2$ (PaCO$_2$ = 20 mmHg approximates 36 mL CO$_2$/100mL blood, and PaCO$_2$ = 80 mmHg approximates 64 mL CO$_2$/100mL blood)

C: compliance; used to describe the change in volume versus change in distending pressure (i.e., ΔV/ΔP), analogous to "distensibility," or the ease with which something can be stretched or distorted

Ctotal or Crs: total respiratory compliance (expressed as mL/cmH$_2$O), which represents the combined elastic load of both the lung (Clung) and the chest wall (Ccw), calculated as 1/Crs, total = 1/Clung + 1/Ccw, for a normal/healthy person at FRC Ctotal (100 mL/cmH$_2$O)

Clung: lung compliance; refers to the slope of the pressure-volume curve obtained during deflation from TLC; normal/healthy value = 200 mL/cmH$_2$O

Cstl: static lung compliance-measurements obtained at zero airflow without lung expansion or movement, calculated with spontaneous breathing as change in volume versus transpulmonary pressure with Ppl estimated by an esophageal balloon and calculated on invasive mechanical ventilation as Vt/(Pplat − end-expiratory pressure), where on mechanical ventilation end-expiratory pressure often equals PEEP

Cstcw: static chest-wall compliance, normal/healthy value = 200 mL/cmH$_2$O

Cldyn: dynamic lung compliance; refers to the ratio of change in volume to change in alveolar distending pressure over a tidal breath with pressure measured at moments of zero flow during the course of active uninterrupted breathing and calculated as the slope of the P-V curve from the beginning to end of a single inspiration

Ccw: chest-wall compliance

CA: carbonic anhydrase; enzyme that catalyzes/accelerates the conversion of CO$_2$ + H$_2$O into carbonic acid

CCHS: central congenital hypoventilation syndrome
CF: cystic fibrosis
CO: cardiac output (L/min)
CO_2: carbon dioxide
COPD: chronic obstructive pulmonary disease
CNS: central nervous system
CPAP: continuous positive airway pressure
CSF: cerebral spinal fluid
CT: computerized tomography
DH: dynamic hyperinflation
DO_2: oxygen delivery; expressed as mL/min or mL/kg/min and measuring approximately 16 mLO_2/kg/min in healthy subjects or 1000 mL O_2/min
DRG: dorsal respiratory group
e: expiratory/expiration
E: elastance; represents the reciprocal of compliance and refers to properties of matter, which allows it to return to its original resting state after being deformed by some external pressure; calculated as $\Delta P/\Delta V$ (cmH_2O/mL) analogous to "stiffness," that is, the tendency to oppose stretch or distortion and revert to original resting configuration
Estl: static lung elastance
Edynl: dynamic lung elastance
Ecw: chest-wall elastance
$ETCO_2$: end-tidal carbon dioxide, usually expressed as a percentage (normal range 4–6%) or in terms on mmHg (normal value for $ETCO_2$ approximating $PaCO_2$ = 40 mmHg)
FEV1: forced expiratory volume in one second
FRC: functional residual capacity; the total volume of air/respirable gas remaining in the lung at end-expiration in the absence of muscle effort, to maintain FRC in healthy subjects usually requires transpulmonary pressure approximately –5 cm H_2O, and in healthy individuals FRC volume measures approximately 36 percent of vital capacity

H^+: proton, i.e., hydrogen ion
H_2O: water
HCO_3^-: bicarbonate ion
H_2CO_3: carbonic acid
Hgb: hemoglobin
HTN: hypertension
I or i: inspiration/inspiratory
ICU: intensive-care unit
Kg: kilogram
KS: kyphoscoliosis
L: liter
LIP: lower inflection point; the transition in volume change of P-V curve from the relatively flat initial portions of lung expansion and the change to the steep hypercompliant phase of the P-V curve—that is, the transition point of the lower portion of the S-shaped sigmoidal P-V curve
mL: milliliter
mmHg: millimeter of mercury
min: minute
MIGET: multiple inert gas elimination technique
mPAP: mean pulmonary arterial pressure
MVO_2: mixed venous oxygen; expressed as either partial pressure (normal value = 40 mmHg) or percent saturation (normal value = 75%)
O_2: oxygen
OHS: obesity hypoventilation syndrome
P0.1: airway occlusion pressure measured at airway opening 0.1 second (100 ms) after initiation of spontaneous breath against an occluded airway, usually measured with an esophageal balloon and expressed as cmH_2O
Ppeak: peak airway pressure
Pplat: plateau airway pressure; the linear phase of the pressure tracing on mechanical ventilation after an inspiratory pause with zero airflow, thought to be reflective of the primary distending pressure to maintain lung inflation at a set volume

Pao: pressure at airway opening
Paw: airway pressure
PA: alveolar pressure
Patm: atmospheric pressure (usually 760 mmHg at sea level)
Ppl: pleural pressure
PaO_2: arterial partial pressure of oxygen
$PaCO_2$: arterial partial pressure of carbon dioxide
Pb: barometric pressure
Pdi: transdiaphragmatic pressure during active contraction, calculated as (Pga − Pes) and often referenced to tidal breathing
Pdimax: maximum transdiaphragmatic pressure, calculated during a maximal inspiratory effort
Pes: esophageal pressure
Pga: gastric pressure
PE: pulmonary embolism
PH: pulmonary hypertension
PAH: pulmonary arterial hypertension
PAP: pulmonary arterial pressure (mPAP = mean PAP); normal values include PAP systolic = 25 mmHg; PAP diastolic = 10 mmHg; mPAP = 15 mmHg
PCWP: pulmonary capillary wedge pressure / pulmonary arterial occlusion pressure; normal values 8 − 12 mmHg
PVR: pulmonary vascular resistance calculated as [(mPAP − PCWP)/CO]
PEEP: positive end-expiratory pressure
$PeCO_2$: expired carbon dioxide pressure
$PACO_2$: alveolar carbon dioxide pressure
P-V: pressure-volume
Q̇: perfusion / blood flow
Q̇s/Q̇t: venous admixture; this value represents an estimation of the volume of gas exchange resulting from an increase in blood flow to the overall shunt compartment of the lungs, where shunt compartment is the sum of the contributions of both true right-to-left shunt + lung units with shuntlike physiology as manifested by units with low V/Q ratios

Raw: airway resistance; calculated from mechanical ventilator parameters as (Ppk − Pplat)/V˙i where V˙i = inspiratory flow rate and expressed as $cmH_2O/L/sec$ with normal values < 1 $cmH_2O/L/sec$
RBC: red blood cell
RV: residual volume; volume of air/gas remaining in the lung/thorax at end of maximal forced expiration
Shunt: that part of lung perfusion that does not participate in gas exchange
Time constant: product of resistance × compliance as expressed as seconds and represents the rapidity or rate of volume change in a specific lung unit or region in response to changes in inflation or deflation pressure
Ti: inspiratory time
Ttot: total respiratory time, both inspiration and expiration, of a single full breathing cycle
Ti/Ttot: duty cycle of the diaphragm used to define the fraction of time during which the diaphragm muscle is actively contracting during a single full breathing cycle
TTdi: tension-time index; calculated as the product of (Pdi/Pdimax × Ti/Ttot)
Tlim: endurance time point at which Pdi can no longer be sustained at a targeted level
TLC: total lung capacity; represents the total volume of air/gas within entire thoracic at maximal/full inspiration and equals the sum of residual volume + inspiratory vital capacity
Ptp: transpulmonary pressure; this pressure represents the total pressure across the lung; i.e., the pressure difference between Pao (airway opening pressure) or Pm (mouth pressure) and pleural pressure (Ppl). Ptp is the sum of three pressure elements: (a) Pel (elastic distending pressure), (b) Pfr (flow resistance pressure), and (c) Pin (inertia). Ptp = (Pao − Palv) − (Palv − Ppl) = Pao − Ppl
Transairway pressure: Pao − Palv, which is the pressure gradient to overcome the resistance to flow down the tracheobronchial tree
Transthoracic lung pressure: Palv − Ppl, which represents the pressure gradient to achieve expansion of the elastic lung component of ventilation

Transthoracic chest wall pressure: Ppl – Patm

Transrespiratory pressure: Pao – Patm, which represents for patients on invasive mechanical ventilation the total positive pressure gradient to generate inspiration—namely, airway + lung + chest wall

UIP: upper inflection point; the transition in volume change at beginning of the relatively flat plateau upper portion of the P-V curve during inspiration thought to represent limits to increased lung expansion due to stiffness/restrictions of the lung collagen matrix/network

UAO: upper-airway obstruction

VC: vital capacity; the total/maximal volume of air/gas available for respiration during inspiration and expiration, which is the volume of air/gas that can be exchanged during the "vital" process of living ventilation

$\dot{V}e$: minute ventilation

$\dot{V}i$: inspiratory flow

Vt: tidal volume; volume of air inspired or expired with each breath during quiet/restful breathing

$\dot{V}$: ventilation

$\dot{V}A$: alveolar ventilation

VTE: venous-thromboembolic disease

V/Q: ventilation perfusion ratio

Vd: dead space; that part of ventilation or tidal volume that does not participate in gas exchange

Vd/Vt: dead space to tidal volume ratio/fraction

Vd(anat): anatomic dead space; fixed volume of the conducting air passages that do not participate in gas exchange (range 150–180 mL)

Vd(phys): physiological dead space; that part of the tidal volume that does not equilibrate with pulmonary blood = Vdanatomic + Vdalveolar

Vd(alv): alveolar dead space; the variable/changing component of total physiological dead space that represents alveoli that are ventilated but not perfused—mathematically, the excess of physiological dead space over the anatomical dead space

$\dot{V}O_2$: total body oxygen consumption

V̇CO$_2$: total body carbon dioxide production
V̇O$_2$resp: oxygen cost of breathing, volume of O$_2$ consumed by the respiratory muscles during active breathing/ventilation
VRG: ventral respiratory group
WOB: work of breathing

Introduction

• • •

For ease of understanding, the **lungs** can be divided anatomically, and in many ways functionally and physiologically, into three main components: (a) the airways (both upper and lower) acting as conduits designed to conduct/transport large volumes of air/respirable gases during both inspiration and expiration distally to and from the (b) parenchyma or gas exchange alveolar-capillary interface consisting of predominately alveolar ducts and alveolar sacs and (c) the pulmonary circulation that eventually transports the end product of either efficient or deficient gas exchange to the systemic circulation. Each of these unique components has specific physiological attributes but also limits that either can preserve health or cause disease.

The architecture of the lung consists of a tubular dichotomous branching structure consisting of twenty to twenty-five branching generations. The first (approximately) sixteen generations consist predominately of the conducting airways, and generations seventeen through twenty-five consist of the gas exchange regions of the lungs, including the respiratory bronchioles, alveolar ducts, and alveolar sacs. However, the entirety of the **respiratory system** consists of multiple additional and intricately intertwined components that encompass the entirety of functions requisite for ventilation and oxygenation. Besides the lung itself, other major components of the respiratory system include (a) the central nervous system (CNS) respiratory neurons (both voluntary and involuntary), (b) the neuroeffector neuromuscular functional system that translates "drive" into effective "mechanical" efforts, and (c) the respiratory system muscles (both inspiratory and expiratory). To put the complexity of respiration in context, measurements of various physiologic parameters and anatomic sites in healthy individuals have revealed astounding numbers, such as that (a) the total number of terminal bronchioles = 22,300 +/- 3,900 per lung (McDonough 2011), (b) the total number of alveoli = mean 480 million (range 274–790) (Ochs 2004), and (c) the daily exchange of approximately 15,000 L of air / respirable gases per day.

Acknowledging the complexity and multiple components of the respiratory system, the primal and evolutionary primary physiological function of the lung is gas exchange—that is, the elimination of vast quantities of carbon dioxide (CO_2) (minimum 288,000 mL/day) produced by body metabolism and the extraction of oxygen (O_2) from the external atmosphere to satisfy the metabolic requirements necessary for healthy organ function and survival (minimum 360,000 mL/day). The gas exchange function of the respiratory system is composed of two distinct but obviously interrelated physiological processes—namely, ventilation and oxygenation.

Ventilation is the elimination of the primary metabolic product of human oxidative metabolism—namely, CO_2. Ventilation involves all components of the respiratory system, including central neurological respiratory drive (both involuntary and voluntary); neuromuscular effector function dependent upon the brainstem connections of the respiratory centers to the spinal cord, the phrenic nerve, the diaphragm (the primary muscle of inspiration), and the chest wall (including the abdomen); plus effective gas-exchange function of the lungs, including the airways, parenchyma, and circulation. The elimination of CO_2 is coupled with (but not totally dependent on) the uptake of oxygen (O_2) from the ambient atmosphere / environmental air for distributions to the metabolizing tissues through the various components of O_2 tissue delivery. Sometimes lost in the gas-exchange function of the lung is the importance of the pulmonary circulation to not only distribute high levels of CO_2 from the metabolizing tissues to the lung for excretion but also regulate ventilation/perfusion ratios at "ideal" levels to guarantee optimal CO_2 elimination and arterial blood oxygenation within the structure of the gas exchange units of the lung itself. Although, in clinical practice, indices of oxygenation tend to dominate the perceptions of lung importance in health and disease; in fact, all aspects of respiratory physiology are vitally and integrally linked. Any understanding of the CO_2/O_2 functions of the respiratory system must first begin with comprehension of the chemical properties and physical characteristics of CO_2 and O_2 themselves as related to content, transport, and homeostasis of each chemical entity.

References

McDonough, J. E., R. Yuan, M. Suzuki, N. Seyednejad, W. M. Elliott, P. G. Sanchez, A. C. Wright, W. B. Gefter, L. Litzky, H. O. Coxson, P. D. Pare, D. D. Sin, R. A. Pierce, J.C. Woods, A. M. McWilliams, J. R. Mayo, S. C. Lam, J. D. Cooper, and J. C. Hogg. 2011. "Small Airway Obstruction and Emphysema in Chronic Obstructive Pulmonary Disease." *New England Journal of Medicine* 365: 1567–1575.

Ochs, M., J. R. Nyengaard, A. Jung, L. Knudson, M. Voigt, T. Wahlers, J. Richter, and H. J. G. Gundersen. 2004. "The Number of Alveoli in the Human Lung." *American Journal of Respiratory and Critical Care Med* 169: 120–124.

CHAPTER 1

Carbon Dioxide (CO_2)

• • •

RESPIRATORY GASES ARE RELATIVELY INSOLUBLE in aqueous solutions, and thus specialized systems have evolved to efficiently transport relatively large volumes of both oxygen (O_2) and carbon dioxide (CO_2) in whole blood. Under both healthy conditions and in relation to many disease states, there exist virtually no limits to the ability of the lungs and the individual alveoli to excrete CO_2. This contrasts with the fixed limits of arterial blood oxygenation; in the healthy lung, the total volume of O_2 uptake is limited by perfusion (i.e., blood flow) and in the circulation by the saturability of its main transport mechanism—namely, binding to hemoglobin (Hgb), contained within red blood cells (RBC). These same principles also apply to disease states whereby well-functioning alveoli can compensate with increased individual alveoli CO_2 elimination in compensation for diseased alveoli with deficient CO_2 excretion within a certain range of magnitude of abnormality to still preserve arterial partial pressure of CO_2 ($PaCO_2$) within the normal range. The same principle cannot be stated for the process of oxygenation in states of lung disease, whereby given the maximal saturability of hemoglobin at 100 percent, any degree of inefficient alveoli oxygenation will always reduce the saturability of the total volume of hemoglobin exiting the pulmonary circulation, resulting in reduced oxygen content subsequently entering the left side of the heart for distribution to the systemic circulation.

Simplistically, but factually also, the lung can be envisioned as a **pump** for CO_2 and a **sump** or **reservoir** for O_2. The daily production of CO_2

approximates 15,000 mmol/day (10.4 mmol/minute), which in turn generates daily acid load of 20×10^6 mEq/day. Normal rates of lung acid (H⁺) excretion approximate 9 mEq/hr, or 13,000 mEq/day, compared to renal/kidney acid (H⁺) excretion of only 40–80 mEq/day. As with virtually every aspect of human metabolism and function, the body has developed unique mechanisms both for the transport of these large quantities of CO_2 and ease of elimination from the circulation without buildup or accumulation of noxious or injurious chemicals. It has also developed mechanisms to maintain a balance between CO_2 production and CO_2 elimination to maintain arterial blood levels of dissolved CO_2 ($PaCO_2$) within a remarkable narrow range; that is, $PaCO_2$ = 40 mmHg +/– 2. This adaptability attests to the high level of integration of the various components of ventilation and also to the adaptability of the lung as a pump and of each individual alveolus to dramatically increase CO_2 elimination based upon metabolic need and resultant alveolar ventilation (V̇A). Surprisingly, it is not the level of arterial CO_2 ($PaCO_2$) per se that serves as the controller molecule/signal to tightly regulate ventilation in response to metabolism but rather the impact of $PaCO_2$ upon the pH or acid (H⁺) content of the cerebral spinal fluid (CSF) that perfuse the lower pons and upper medulla central nervous system (CNS) respiratory centers—most specifically, the intracellular pH (pHi) of individual neurons located in the inspiratory center.

The importance of the CO_2 transport mechanisms not only relates to CO_2 homeostasis and maintenance of $PaCO_2$ within a very narrow range but also provides an efficient blood and tissue buffering system to mitigate deleterious effects upon both arterial blood and total body acid base status / hemostasis (i.e., pH). In relation to CO_2, this is especially important given this large acid load whereby the most important nonbicarbonate buffers in the body are proteins (especially hemoglobin) and, to a lesser extent, phosphates and ammonium. These massive volumes of CO_2 diffuse from metabolizing tissues into the venous circulation for subsequent transport to the lung for elimination. Once released from the tissues during oxidative metabolism, CO_2 transport in the blood occurs in two distinct forms:

CO_2 transported in plasma and CO_2 transported within the RBC (Guyton 1982, Figure 28-12; West 2005, Figure 6-5).

Under resting conditions and in health, the total body CO_2 production ($\dot{V}eCO_2$) approximates 200 mL/min, as determined by measurements of expiratory gas concentrations and volumes. In disease states associated with high metabolic catabolism or high degrees of tissue damage, the $\dot{V}eCO_2$ can increase to levels double the resting healthy state. However the extremes of $\dot{V}eCO_2$ are most evident upon exercise with values in highly conditioned athletes measured at 6 L/min. Even at these high levels of metabolism, the entirety of the respiratory systems is remarkably efficient at maintaining $PaCO_2$ within the normal range. This remarkable efficiency is reflected by the fact that the diffusion capacity of the lung for CO_2 is so great that it cannot currently be accurately measured in humans in vivo.

Table 1.1: Contribution of Different Pathways to CO_2 Transport and Exchange (Klocke 1991)

	Arterial Content	
	mL/dL blood	Percent of total
Plasma		
Dissolved CO_2	1.51	3.1%
Bicarbonate	30.01	62.1%
Carbamate	0.67	1.4%
Total CO_2 content	32.19	66.6%
Erythrocyte (RBC)		
Dissolved CO_2	0.93	1.9%
Bicarbonate	12.58	26.0%
Carbamate	2.67	5.5%
Total CO_2 content	16.18	33.4%

When present in solution, CO_2 combines with water (H_2O) to generate carbonic acid (H_2CO_3) that dissociates almost instantaneously to free H^+ and bicarbonate anion (HCO_3^-), which reaction is rapidly accelerated in the presence of the enzyme carbonic anhydrase (CA). A similar chemical reaction occurs within the RBC as CO_2 also rapidly diffuses across the RBC membrane and, since intracellular RBCs possess carbonic anhydrase, such that each single RBC (erythrocyte) can individually accelerate the chemical metabolism of CO_2. Thus the RBC functions as a key intermediate (i.e., middleman) in total-body CO_2 transport. As CO_2 diffuses from metabolizing tissues into whole blood, it passes freely into RBCs, where carbonic anhydrase (CA) rapidly accelerates its hydration to carbonic acid (H_2CO_3). As carbonic acid content of the RBC increases, it dissociates almost instantaneously into H^+ and HCO_3^-. Equimolar amounts of HCO_3^- then diffuse into the venous blood, making the total contribution of CO_2 buffering capacity as HCO_3^- approximately 70–80 percent. The HCO_3^- generated by this reaction freely diffuses into the plasma, and to maintain electrical neutrality, an equivalent concentration of chloride anion moves into the red blood cells, termed the "chloride shift."

Hemoglobin contained within the RBC is also able to buffer CO_2 over the entirety of the physiological pH range almost exclusively by forming carbamino-hemoglobin (carbamate) through binding with the nine histidine residues on each of the four polypeptde chains of hemoglobin. Approximately 10–20 percent of the total body CO_2 load is transported as carbamino-hemoglobin (carbamate) restrained within the RBC. Carbamate represents the salt of carbamic acid formed by the reaction of CO_2 with certain amino acids of the hemoglobin molecule as CO_2 and H^+ reversibly bind to uncharged amino groups of the protein carbamic acid. The affinity of Hgb for H^+ rapidly buffers the free acid, whose buffering capacity is actually enhanced at the reduced pO_2 values in venous blood.

The remainder of total-body CO_2 transport exists in whole blood in free dissolved state (i.e., $PaCO_2$), noting the solubility of CO_2 in water at 37ºC = 0.06 $mLCO_2$/dL/mmHg. Only approximately 5–8 percent of the daily CO_2 load is transported in blood/plasma as dissolved CO_2 ($PaCO_2$), which you will note is actually much higher in comparison to dissolved O_2 in arterial blood (whose value approximates 2%), noting that the solubility of O_2 in water at 37°C = 0.003 mL O_2/dL/mmHg.

Thus the majority of CO_2 is transported in whole blood (including both the plasma and RBC components) as HCO_3^- through the action of carbonic anhydrase (approximately 70–80%). The total blood bicarbonate content then consists of the serum/plasma bicarbonate concentration plus the amount of dissolved CO_2, calculated as 0.06 mL/ 100 mL blood × $PaCO_2$. In absolute terms, the arterial CO_2 content ($CaCO_2$) approximates 36 mL CO_2/100mL blood at $PaCO_2$ = 20 mmHg; 50 mL CO_2/100 mL blood at $PaCO_2$ = 40 mmHg, and 64 mL CO_2/100mL blood at PaCO2 = 80 mmHg (Guyton 1982; Tisi 1983).

As venous blood enters the alveolar bed, dissolved CO_2 (venous CO_2 partial pressure approximately 46 mmHg) is excreted almost instantaneously as blood enters the alveolar-capillary bed, but it constitutes only at most 8 percent of the total quantity of CO_2 exchanged during capillary transit. The majority of excreted CO_2 enters the pulmonary capillary bed as bicarbonate ion (HCO_3^-) generated predominately by the catalytic activity of carbonic anhydrase. As dissolved CO_2 leaves the alveolar capillary blood and diffuses across the interstitial space and across type II epithelial pneumocytes for subsequent excretion, this equilibration is disturbed, leading to further production of CO_2 converted from the high-concentration of HCO_3^- (70–80%) entering the alveolar-capillary bed, which also rapidly diffuses across the alveolar-capillary bed for effective high-volume elimination of CO_2. This chemical reaction continues indefinitely to maintain a constant highly effective continual elimination of CO_2 (West 2005: Figure 6-5). Thus in effect, CO_2 elimination across the alveolar-capillary membrane of the lung is the exact opposite of the chemical reactions that loads CO_2 from metabolizing tissues into whole blood and the RBC.

In contrast to oxygen saturation, the saturability of hemoglobin with CO_2 is relatively linear, ensuring the effectiveness of the acid buffering capacity of the RBC. The CO_2 dissociation curve describes the summed contributions of all pathways of CO_2 transport as a function of CO_2 tension / partial pressure. The CO_2 dissociation curve is relatively steep (especially within the normal physiological range) in comparison to the O_2 dissociation curve; consequently, large volumes of CO_2 can be exchanged with relatively small alterations in blood $PaCO_2$. The steep slope of the CO_2 dissociation curve permits the continuous excretion of CO_2, albeit with less efficiency in disease states associated with abnormal distributions of pulmonary ventilation (V) and blood flow (Q). In contrast, O_2 exchange is more susceptible to alterations in V/Q matching or mismatching (West 2005, Figures 6-6 and 6-7).

In summary, the majority of $\dot{V}eCO_2$ is transported in blood as HCO_3^-, with the RBC functioning as a major source of transport and buffering capacity for most of the daily CO_2 production and consequent total-body acid load. Although CO_2 has an aqueous solubility twenty times that of O_2, CO_2 dissolved in physical state accounts for only 5–7 percent of total blood CO_2 content of arterial and venous blood. Nevertheless, dissolved CO_2 plays a pivotal role in CO_2 transport and exchange by providing ready access of substrate for bicarbonate and carbamate pools. Besides providing a remarkably efficient buffering system that maintains arterial blood pH within a very narrow range (normal pH = 7.40 +/- 0.02), this system also ensures a continuous gradient for efficient removal of dissolved CO_2 ($PaCO_2$) by the lungs and respiratory system at the alveolar level. The multiple chemical reactions that consume these large amounts of CO_2 allow for both efficient buffering of a high acid load and a favorable alveolar-capillary CO_2 gradient for ease of lung removal and elimination.

REFERENCES

Guyton, A. C. 1982. "Transport of Oxygen and Carbon Dioxide between the Alveoli and Tissue Cells." In *Human Physiology and Mechanisms of Disease*. Philadelphia: W. B. Saunders Company. 305–317.

Klocke, R. A. 1991. "Carbon Dioxide." In *The Lung Scientific Foundations*, edited by R. G. Crystal and J. B. West. New York: Raven Press. 1233–1239.

Tisi, G.M. 1983. "Clinical Physiology." In *Pulmonary Physiology in Clinical Medicine*. Baltimore: Williams & Wilkins. 3–28.

West, J. B. 2005. "Gas Transport by the Blood." In *Respiratory Physiology: The Essentials*. Philadelphia: Wolters Kluwer/Lippincott Williams & Wilkins. 75–89.

CHAPTER 2

Oxygen (O_2)

• • •

JUST AS THE RED BLOOD cell (RBC) is a key component and important intermediary in the transport of carbon dioxide (CO_2), the RBC is even more important as virtually the sole vital transporter of oxygen (O_2). Any understanding of oxygen transport/balance must first begin with a clear understanding of the oxygen-hemoglobin (O_2-Hgb) dissociation curve and its importance in maximizing whole blood oxygen carrying capacity (i.e., arterial oxygen content [CaO_2]), especially given the relatively low solubility of oxygen dissolved in blood (0.003 mL/dL/mmHg) but also as related to both uptake of oxygen at the alveolar level and its transport and subsequent release to metabolizing tissues. Hemoglobin (Hgb) consists of heme (an iron porphyrin compound) and a protein (globin) that has four polypeptide chains. Four molecules of oxygen can bind with each molecule of Hgb, and further binding of O_2 to one Hgb moiety facilitates the binding to the remaining three heme rings of the tetrameric Hgb molecule. The relationship between the partial pressure of oxygen and the number of binding sites of Hgb that have O_2 attached is known as the oxygen-Hgb dissociation curve (Snyder 1987, Figure 1-2; West 2012, Figure 6-1).

The memorization of some key physiologically significant numbers and values evident under healthy conditions can easily allow for a rough drafting of this relationship: (a) the p50 of hemoglobin—that being the PaO_2, at which hemoglobin is 50 percent saturated, is 27 mmHg; (b) the values reflective of mixed venous blood in health (MVO_2 = 40 mmHg/

percent saturation = 75%); (c) PaO_2 = 60 mmHg equivalent to approximately 90 percent saturation; and (d) normal values for arterial blood (PaO_2 = 100 mmHg/100% saturation) (Crapo 1999). As is obvious from review of any figure or graphic characteristics of the O_2-Hgb dissociation curve, the shape is nonlinear; in fact, it is S-shaped or curvilinear in configuration. Beside the correlative values of PaO_2 and Hgb percent saturation, a number of additional very important physiological principles can also be ascertained from review of the O_2-Hgb curve: (a) the relatively steep increase in oxygen saturation and thus blood oxygen loading at values above the tissue level (i.e., MVO_2 = 40 mmHg); until (b) plateau in oxygen saturation is reached beginning at PaO_2 = 60 mmHg, which corresponds to approximately 90 percent hemoglobin saturation, which then peaks at 100 percent at values approximately 100 mmHg; and (c) the inability to increase hemoglobin saturation at values above 100 percent, regardless of increases in inspired oxygen concentration/fraction (FiO_2) or magnitude of PaO_2 (West 2005, Figure 6-1).

At the tissue level, the steep portion of the O_2-Hgb dissociation curve also allows for large volumes of O_2 to be released to metabolizing tissues while (a) still maintaining a relatively high saturation and O_2 carriage (i.e., O_2 reserve) and (b) still maintaining relatively steep partial-pressure gradient between systemic capillary blood and metabolizing tissues. The relatively flat portion of the O_2-Hgb dissociation curve at 100 percent saturation has two important physiological principles: (a) from a positive perspective, at room air (FiO_2 = 21%) decrements in PaO_2 of 20–30 mmHg can be well tolerated without appreciable decreases in O_2 percent saturation and consequently CaO_2; and (b) just as important, at the alveolar-capillary level where oxygen uptake occurs, a relatively large partial-pressure gradient for soluble O_2 diffusion will always be maintained between the alveolus and capillary blood/plasma, even when most of the O_2 is loaded to Hgb. This physiological design or evolutionary adaptation functions to maintain adequate levels of oxygen transport by hemoglobin within the range of ambient-inspired oxygen concentrations while enhancing release into metabolizing tissues where tissue-venous oxygen tension approaches values less than 40 mmHg. At the metabolizing tissue level, Hgb can then release approximately 25–30 percent of the total blood oxygen load / carrying capacity (approximate normal value of oxygen extraction in health).

As expected, various clinical conditions can modify the characteristics of the O_2-Hgb dissociation curve to assist in meeting tissue demands at any given circumstance. If O_2 affinity for Hgb increases, the O_2-Hgb dissociation curve shifts to the left, and if O_2 affinity for Hgb decreases, this curve is shifted to the right. In addition, under conditions of increased tissue metabolic needs, as may be evident under conditions of anaerobic cellular metabolism and metabolic acidosis, the O_2-Hgb dissociation curve is shifted to the right to allow greater "unloading" of oxygen at the tissue level to increase O_2 utilization, perhaps even in the absence of changes in tissue perfusion (i.e., for any given PaO_2, the percent saturation is lower, and thus percent binding strength is lower, allowing for more O_2 to freely diffuse into the highly metabolically active tissues). The chemical entity 2-3 diphosphoglycerate (2-3DPG) is an end product of RBC metabolism, which increases under conditions of chronic hypoxia, which also causes the O_2-Hgb curve to shift to the right, again assisting in unloading oxygen at tissue level when O_2 delivery is reduced (West 2012, Figure 6-3). Systemic alkalosis shifts this curve in the opposite direction (Snyder 1987, Figure 1-4).

As expected, the rate of O_2 uptake across the alveolar precapillary arterioles and capillaries is not linear or constant. In pulmonary arterioles, O_2 saturation levels increase exponentially with decreasing vessel diameter. Oxygen saturation levels remain relatively stable along the feeding pulmonary arterioles until RBC has reached the precapillary arterioles, and from that point on, rapid O_2 uptake occurs. Once the RBC has entered capillaries, then the rate of O_2 uptake is slowed. The progressive decline in O_2 uptake rate is consistent with the dependence of the blood-diffusing capacity upon O_2 saturation and the decreased alveolar-vascular O_2 gradient driving O_2 diffusion and uptake along the length of each vascular gas exchange unit. It should also be noted that pulmonary blood flow velocity is also not linear or constant across the full circulation of the lung but slows appreciably as it enters the capillary bed (Tabuchi 2013, Figure 3).

The remarkable ability of Hgb to bind, transport, and release molecules of O_2 efficiently, dependent upon physiological need/demand, allows for the utilization of large quantities of O_2 that would *not* be available through dissolved O_2 alone. This distinction is exemplified by analyses of the various components that constitute the arterial oxygen content (CaO_2 = O_2 dissolved in plasma + O_2 hemoglobin bound), which in purely mathematical terms can be calculated as CaO_2 = 0.003 mL (PaO_2) + (1.39 mLO_2/100 mL blood × [Hgb gm/mL] × % hemoglobin oxygen saturation). Under healthy conditions, CaO_2 = 20 mL/100 mL blood (Hgb bound) + 0.3 mL/100 mL blood (dissolved); approximately 20.3 vol% (Snyder 1987). It is quite obvious, based upon this equation, that well over 95 percent of oxygen transported in blood represents oxygen bound to hemoglobin; and in normal, nondiseased, healthy situations, it equals approximately 20 mLO_2/100 mL blood but only 0.003 mLO_2/100 mL dissolved in blood per mmHg. At normal values of PaO_2 = 100 at total of 0.3 mLO_2/100 mL, blood is dissolved in plasma during healthy conditions. This dissolved O_2 component of CaO_2 represents only approximately 2 percent of the total CaO_2 content, which is far less than the dissolved CO_2 represented component of $CaCO_2$.

Just as importantly, in relation to the care of critically ill patients, an understanding of the components and concepts of oxygen delivery (DO_2) is vital to maintaining adequate tissue vitality and avoiding ischemic injury or tissue necrosis. Similar to dissolved O_2 representing a relatively low magnitude of CaO_2, in relation to O_2 delivery, CaO_2 represents a relatively smaller but still important component of DO_2 compared to cardiac output. The components of DO_2 = CO × CaO_2 again note that by far the cardiac output (CO) or, more specifically, individual tissue perfusion is a much greater component of DO_2 than CaO_2, and in a vast majority of clinical scenarios, it is the failure of global CO or focal tissue perfusion rather than decreases in CaO_2 that results in ischemic organ damage (Snyder 1987).

Organ-specific tissue blood perfusion, capillary oxygen extraction, and oxygen uptake or consumption are uniquely linked to the particular metabolic functions and survival of each individual organ (Gorlin 1978, Figure 8-4). As an example, the kidneys receive a relatively large proportion of the overall body CO to satisfy their physiological functions of blood purification but have relatively low values of oxygen consumption, thus causing blood flow to leave the kidney on the venous side with a relatively high oxygen saturation and content. It is for this reason that the oxygen saturation of the inferior vena cava slightly exceeds that of the superior vena cava (Nelson 1987; Evans 2008; Gardiner 2011). Conversely, the heart requires a relatively large volume of oxygen extraction (high extraction fraction) through its capillary system, and thus venous blood exiting the metabolizing tissues of the heart into the cardiac sinuses and veins has a relatively low level of oxygen saturation and content, approximating 20 mmHg (30% oxygen saturation), which represents the lowest values for venous oxygen in health throughout the entire body (Gorlin 1978, Figure 8-4).

Acknowledging the importance of regional and tissue-specific O_2 requirements, in general, critical-care medicine has focused only upon total body indices of oxygenation parameters to assess tissue viability and monitor and/or adjust care heavily weighted by the focus upon sepsis and septic shock. Analyses of samples of arterial blood for oxygen saturation and content plus analyses of samples of blood recovered from the proximal port of a pulmonary arterial catheter, which represent blood returning to the right ventricle of the heart from both the inferior and superior vena cavae (thus termed mixed venous blood) when associated with simultaneous measurements of CO, allow for the calculation of a variety of indices relating to the effectiveness or lack of effectiveness of overall total body oxygen delivery, tissue extraction, and O_2 utilization. Understanding the normal values and, subsequently, the abnormal values for these measurements then allows potential to therapeutically manipulate various variables to improve tissue DO_2 and potentially improve patient outcome.

Table 2.1: Resting Measurements of Tissue-Specific Oxygen (O_2) Delivery and Utilization

	Total/Systemic	Renal/Kidney	Cardiac/Heart
O_2 Delivery (mL/min)	640–1200	128–240	40–45
O_2 Consumption (mL/min)	180–280	25	30
O_2 Extraction Fraction	22–30%	10%	55–70%
Venous pO_2 (mmHg)	40	50	18–20
Venous % Saturation	75%	83%	30%

REFERENCES

Crapo, R. O., R. L. Jensen, M. Hegewald, and D. P. Tashkin. 1999. "Arterial Blood Gas Reference Values for Sea Level and at Altitude of 1,400 Meters." *American Journal of Respiratory and Critical Care Medicine* 160: 1525–1531.

Evans, R. G., B. S. Gardiner, D. W. Smith, and P. M. O'Connor. 2008. "Intrarenal Oxygenation: Unique Challenges and the Biophysical Basis of Homeostasis." *American Journal of Physiology: Renal Physiology* 295: F1259–F1270.

Gardiner, B. S., D. W. Smith, P. M. O'Connor, and R. G. Evans. 2011. "A Mathematical Model of Diffusional Shunting of Oxygen from Arteries to Veins in the Kidney." *American Journal of Physiology: Renal Physiology* 300: F1339–F1352.

Gorlin, R., and M. V. Herman. 1978. Physiology of the Coronary Circulation. In *The Heart*, edited by J. W. Hurst. New York: McGraw-Hill Book Company. 101–106.

Nelson, L. D. 1987. "Oxygen Transport: The Model and Reality." In *Oxygen Transport in the Critically Ill*, edited by J. V. Snyder and M. R. Pinsky. Chicago: Year Book Medical Publishers, Inc. 235–248.

Snyder, J. V. 1987. "Oxygen Transport: The Model and Reality." In *Oxygen Transport in the Critically Ill*, edited by J. V. Snyder and M. R. Pinsky. Chicago: Year Book Medical Publishers, Inc. 3–15.

Tabuchi, A., B. Styp-Rekowska, A. S. Slutsky, P. D. Wagner, A. R. Pries, and W. M. Kuebler. 2013. "Precapillary Oxygenation Contributes Relevantly to Gas Exchange in the Intact Lung." *American Review of Respiratory Disease* 188 (4): 474–481.

West, J. B. 2012. "Gas Transport by the Blood." In *Respiratory Physiology: The Essentials*. Philadelphia: Wolters Kluwer/Lippincott Williams & Wilkins. 77–94.

CHAPTER 3
Pulmonary Gas Exchange

• • •

THE ANATOMIC STRUCTURES CONSIDERED TO represent the gas-exchanging portions of the lung exist distal to the terminal bronchioles, sequentially anatomically divided into respiratory bronchioles, alveolar ducts, and alveolar sacs. However, the vast majority of gas exchange, both oxygen (O_2) and carbon dioxide (CO_2), occurs at the alveolar level, consisting of the single layer of capillary endothelial cells, the minuscule interstitial space, and the single-cellular alveolar epithelial cell surface composed predominately of type I alveolar cells/pneumocytes. Given the efficiency of alveolar gas diffusion, pulmonary end-capillary blood/gas partial pressure exactly reflects alveolar gas composition. Again, remembering that the solubility of CO_2 in water is twenty times greater than the solubility of O_2, all gas transport at the pulmonary capillary level occurs through passive diffusion. This difference in solubility far outweighs the slightly smaller molecular size of O_2 in relation to diffusional transport across the alveolar space. Thus CO_2 transport across the alveolar membrane is twenty times greater than the transfer of O_2 when both gases diffuse under the same partial pressure. Therefore a much greater alveolar-capillary PO_2 gradient is required to maintain O_2 transport approximately equal to CO_2.

As previously noted, in the healthy lung, O_2 diffusional transport remains remarkably efficient with near total equilibration across the alveolar membrane occurring within a relatively finite but rapid time frame of

0.25–0.3 seconds, which is well below the average transit time that a single RBC remains within and transverse the alveolar-capillary bed (i.e., 0.5–0.8 seconds), thus accentuating the perfusional (not diffusional) limitation of maximal O_2 uptake at the alveolar capillary level under healthy conditions. In contrast to O_2, the capacitance of CO_2 in the alveolar membrane is sufficient to permit rapid equilibration of CO_2 across this barrier that cannot be measured in vivo.

Given these physical characteristics of both O_2 and CO_2, deleterious abnormalities in pulmonary gas exchange for either CO_2 (hypercapnia) or O_2 (hypoxemia) rarely result from diffusional barrier abnormalities or diffusional impairment but more commonly result from disturbances in the balance of ventilation (V) compared to perfusion (Q) within each individual alveolar unit—namely, ventilation/perfusion (V/Q) ratio inequalities (V/Q mismatch) (West 1977; Wagner 1991). However, regional differences exist even in the healthy lung in relation to the distribution of various V/Q relationships throughout the entire distribution of the whole lung, dependent on and influenced by gravity, lung weight, and the topographic inequality of blood flow based upon regional variations in pulmonary artery pressure, pulmonary alveolar pressure, and pulmonary venous pressure with variable zones of differing ventilation and perfusion relationships. Consequently, in subsequent discussions of gas-exchange abnormalities, especially in relation to specific disease states, the importance of the "dispersion" (actual splay/range of V/Q distributions) of these V/Q ratios throughout the entire lung will become evident (West 1977; West 2005, Figures 5-8 and 5-9). In healthy individuals, V/Q measurements actually represent a range of values whereby 95 percent of both blood flow and ventilation range between V/Q ratios of 0.3–2.1 (Wagner 1974).

Given the chemical and physiological characteristics of O_2 and CO_2, within any gas exchange unit of the lung, partial pressure of oxygen (pO_2), partial pressure of carbon dioxide (pCO_2), and partial pressure of nitrogen (pN_2) are uniquely determined by three major factors: (a) V/Q ratios, (b) composition of inspired gas, and (c) composition of mixed venous blood. Local alveolar PAO_2 and $PACO_2$ and resultant end-capillary O_2 and CO_2 tensions are uniquely set by the local V/Q ratio for a given set of boundary conditions (i.e., the inspired and venous blood composition) and the particular characteristics of the O_2 and CO_2 dissociation curves (West 1977). While breathing room air, these boundary values for inspired pO_2 = 150 mmHg and pCO_2 = 0 mmHg; while respective values for venous tensions reflect mixed venous pO_2 = 40 mmHg and pCO_2 = 45 mmHg. From purely a gas-exchange perspective and under ambient conditions, dependent upon the specific V/Q relationship all potential combinations of pO_2 and pCO_2 will fall within these boundaries, noting every measurement will have a unique single value for pO_2 and pCO_2. For an ideal V/Q = 1, pO_2 = 100 mmHg and pCO_2 = 40 mmHg

Regardless of the direction of V/Q abnormality deviation from the "ideal" value for gas exchange of V/Q = 1 (West 2005, Figure 5-13; Wagner 2009, Figure 3), abnormalities of gas exchange will occur, but the multifold higher dissociation of CO_2 compared to O_2 renders O_2 much more susceptible to develop significant hypoxemia at low V/Q ratios than CO_2 in relation to development of hypercapnia and high V/Q. In relation to efficiency of oxygenation, analysis of end-capillary oxygen content in relation to specific V/Q values demonstrates a steep portion of this curvilinear relationship that is evident within the range and dispersion of V/Q relationships considered within the normal range (0.3 – 2.1) but relatively flat at V/Q values below 0.2 (i.e., end-capillary gas content approaching venous blood composition) and also relatively flat at V/Q values above 10 (i.e., approaching inspired gas composition), thus explaining the higher susceptibility to hypoxemia created by lung units with shunt or shunt-like physiology (West 1991, Figure 2 and Figure 3; West 2005, Figure 2). Analysis of end-capilary pO2 throughout the range of V/Q distributions from zero to infinity demonstrates that as V/Q increases from a value = 0, there is little change from venous values (approximate 40 mmHg) until V/Q = 0.2, then as noted a marked increase in pO2 until V/Q approximates 10 again above which minimal further increase in pO2 is noted.

Thus, the principal effects of V/Q inequality as they apply to CO_2 and O_2 exchange can be summarized as (a) both $PaCO_2$ and PaO_2 are adversely affected no matter what pathological basis for V/Q inequality, (b) V/Q abnormalities will cause alterations in both $PaCO_2$ and PaO_2 but more severe for hypoxemia than hypercapnia, (c) very low regions of V/Q affect O_2 more than CO_2 (with V/Q = 0 representing true anatomic shunt), (d) very high levels of V/Q affect CO_2 more than O_2 (with V/Q = infinity representing pure dead space ventilation), and (e) abnormalities of V/Q increase alveolar-arterial differences for both CO_2 and O_2.

Throughout the discussion of pulmonary gas exchange and mechanisms of hypoxemia and hypercapnia, references will continually be made to the physiological assessment measure of multiple inert gas elimination technique (MIGET) for the following reasons: (a) providing the basis for objectifications of all V/Q relationships data both in health and disease and (b) providing convenient graphics (which can be located in specifically noted references), again as an objective display to assist comprehension of abnormal gas exchange in multiple disease states. MIGET, developed in the 1970s, measures the pulmonary exchange of a set of six different inert gases (SF6, ethane, cyclopropane, enflurane, ether, acetone) dissolved together in solution and infused intravenously. An inert gas is defined as a gas whose transport in the blood is governed only by its physically dissolving chemical (solubility) characteristics. When an inert gas dissolved in saline is steadily infused into the venous circulation, the proportion of gas that is eliminated by ventilation from the blood of any given lung unit depends only on the solubility of the gas and the ventilation-perfusion ratio. These inert gases in solution are then infused intravenously at a constant rate proportional to the minute ventilation. The concentrations of these six inert gases are then measured by gas chromatography in arterial, mixed venous, and mixed-expired exhaled samples, along with a standard arterial blood gas (ABG), and analyzed by computer to generate graphic displays of volumes of both ventilation and blood flow based upon various rates of retention and excretion of each individual inert gas as expressed on the vertical axis in relation of a spectrum of V/Q ratios displayed on the horizontal axis (West 1991, Figure 6 and Figure 8; Melot 1994; Wagner 2009).

Table 3.1: Multiple Inert Gas Elimination Technique (MIGET) Definition of Terms

Shunt	V/Q < 0.005
Low V/Q	0.005 < V/Q < 0.1
High V/Q	10 < V/Q < 100
Dead Space	V/Q > 100

REFERENCES

Melot, C. 1994. "Ventilation-Perfusion Relationships in Acute Respiratory Failure." *Thorax* 49: 1251–1258.

Wagner, P. D, R. B. Laravuso, R. R. Uhl, and J. B. West. 1972. "Continuous Distributions of Ventilation-Perfusion Ratios in Normal Subjects Breathing Air and 100% O_2." *Journal of Clinical Investigation* 54: 54–68.

Wagner, P. D. 2009. "The Multiple Inert Gas Elimination Technique (MIGET)." In *Applied Physiology in Intensive Care Medicine*, edited by M. R. Pinsky, L. Brochard, J. Mancebo, and G. Hedenstierna. Dordrecht: Springer. 29–36.

Wagner, P. D., and R. Rodriguez-Roisin. 1991. "State of Art/Conference Report: Clinical Advances in Pulmonary Gas Exchange." *American Review of Respiratory Disease* 143: 883–888.

West, J. B. 1977. "Ventilation-Perfusion Relationships." *American Review of Respiratory Disease* 116: 919–943.

West, J. B. 2005. "Ventilation Perfusion Relationships." In *Respiratory Physiology: The Essentials*. Philadelphia: Wolters Kluwer/Lippincott Williams & Wilkins. 55–74.

West, J. B., and P. D. Wagner. 1991. "Ventilation Perfusion Relationships." In *The Lung Scientific Foundations*, edited by R. G. Crystal, 1289–1305. New York: Raven Press.

CHAPTER 4

Hypercapnia

• • •

WITHIN THE LUNG THERE ARE obligate areas of ventilation that do not participate in gas exchange for either O_2 or CO_2. From a physiological perspective, these areas are referred to as wasted or dead-space ventilation. The overall total wasted ventilation (termed physiological dead space = Vdphys) is further subdivided into fixed and variable dead-space components as exemplified by the following equation: Vd physiological = Vd anatomic + Vd alveolar. Mechanical ventilation often poses an additional component to Vd because of parts of the ventilator equipment and apparatus.

Anatomic dead-space ventilation (Vdanat) represents the fixed component of wasted ventilation. In an adult, this obligatory anatomic dead space approximates 150–180 mL (approximately 1 mL/pound ideal body weight) that is required to move volumes of air into and out of the large conducting airways, which are devoid of gas exchange capabilities (West 1988). This fixed obligatory anatomic dead space encompasses approximately 50 percent above the carina and 50 percent below the carina. The variable (nonfixed) degree of wasted ventilation that varies from disease to disease is termed the alveolar dead-space ventilation (Vdalv), always representing some degree of alveolar gas exchange inefficiency.

Even under healthy, nondisease conditions, a significant component of every breath does not participate in gas exchange (i.e., wasted ventilation). For convenience the magnitude of wasted ventilation is usually expressed as the ratio of tidal volume (Vt)—namely, dead space to tidal volume ratio/fraction (Vd/Vt) that even under healthy, normal conditions amounts to approximately 30 percent. However, given the relatively high solubility of CO_2 in blood and the anatomic characteristics and physiological efficiency of the alveolar-capillary bed, at the alveolar level, the difference between arterial partial pressure of carbon dioxide ($PaCO_2$) and alveolar pressure of carbon dioxide ($PACO_2$) is relatively small—less than 5 mmHg. In addition, under healthy conditions, end-tidal expired CO_2 ($ETCO_2$) is thought to be equal to $PACO_2$. However, as ventilatory efficiency worsens, both at the individual alveoli level and then at whole lung level, the differences between expired CO_2 ($PECO_2$) and alveolar $PACO_2$ widens, and Vd/Vt increases by the Bohr modification of the Enghoff-Meyer equation (Vd/Vt = $[PACO_2 - PECO_2]/PACO_2$) (Holets 2006).

Simply stated, Vd/Vt measures the efficiency of pulmonary ventilation based upon CO_2 elimination by the lung in comparison to normal healthy, nondiseased lungs. Again, even in situations of lung disease, given the relative nonsaturability of CO_2 elimination, the near linearity of the CO_2 dissociation curve, and the ability to increase minute ventilation ($\dot{V}e$) in response to increase CO_2 loads, this worsening CO_2 elimination or worsening ventilatory efficacy can be accommodated to preserve $PaCO_2$ at normal levels. However, a point is reached at approximately 60 percent Vd/Vt whereby compensatory mechanisms fail and overt hypercapnia ensues. In clinical lung disease, the predominate determinant of worsening Vd/Vt is contributed to by individual alveoli with high V/Q relationships (V/Q > 100). The effects of worsening degrees of Vd/Vt elevation is evident upon review of the curve describing the relationship between $PACO_2$ and alveolar ventilation ($\dot{V}A$), noting the transition point at each level of alveolar ventilation ($\dot{V}A$) whereby hypercapnia develops. Thus, from a lung perspective, independent of abnormalities in CNS respiratory drive, neuroeffector function, and total body CO_2 production ($\dot{V}eCO_2$), elevations in dead-space fraction (Vd/Vt) are the main physiological determinate of clinical hypercapnia (Berger 1988, Figure 7-1).

Simplistically, $PaCO_2$ is linearly related to CO_2 production ($\dot{V}eCO_2$) and inversely related to alveolar ventilation ($\dot{V}A$) as represented by the following mathematical equation: $PaCO_2 = K\ \dot{V}eCO_2/\dot{V}A$ (alveolar ventilation) = K V̇eCO$_2$/V̇e [1 − Vd/Vt], whereby V̇e represents minute ventilation and Vd/Vt represents the proportional fraction of the tidal volume that represents wasted ventilation that does not participate in any way in gas exchange, also referred to as dead-space fraction. As previously noted, even though this equation seems to support a straight linear relationship between V̇A and PaCO$_2$, this relationship is actually curvilinear, whereby there exists a relatively flat portion at higher levels of V̇A with little effect upon decreases in PaCO$_2$ (respiratory alkalosis), but even more importantly, especially as relates to disease states whereby hypercapnia becomes the dominant pathological gas exchange process, there exists a break point whereby once overt hypercapnia becomes manifest, then relatively minor decreases in V̇A will elicit large increases in PaCO$_2$. This exponential relationship of V̇A and PaCO$_2$ at levels of V̇A below normal ventilation is common to many physiological functions and generates a relatively simplistic but important clinical corollary—namely, that relatively large degrees of physiological deterioration are necessary to cause initial yet clinically significant physiological abnormalities (such as the initial development of mild levels of hypercapnia). However, once abnormal and hypercapnia becomes overt, even relatively trivial/minor worsening in ventilatory function will result in dramatic worsening in PaCO$_2$ deteriorations.

The understanding of any clinical condition associated with either hypocapnia or hypercapnia can be ascertained through review of the various individual components of this equation: PaCO$_2$ = K V̇eCO$_2$/V̇A (alveolar ventilation) = K V̇eCO$_2$/V̇e (1 − Vd/Vt), whereby K = 0.863. Increase in PaCO$_2$ will result mathematically by any factors that either increase the numerator and/or decrease the denominator. In health, muscular exercise and associated physical activity or exertion remain the dominate factor for increased V̇eCO$_2$. However, in disease conditions associated with marked hypercatabolism, such as thyrotoxicosis, sepsis, or severe burns, or in patients with coexistent lung disease and restrictions in ventilation receiving excessive quantities of carbohydrate nutritional support can affect a significant increase in V̇eCO$_2$ above the normal resting value of approximately

200 mL/minute. However, as long as V̇A can effectively increase to match the increase in CO_2 delivery to the lung, $PaCO_2$ will remain within the normal range—again remembering the remarkable ability of functional individual alveoli for effective CO_2 elimination.

On the bottom side of this equation ($PaCO_2$ = K V̇eCO_2/V̇e [1 − Vd/Vt]), any factors that decrease V̇e below levels necessary to match oxidative metabolism and/or that increase the dead-space fraction above a threshold level will result in hypercapnia. However, as previously noted, given the linearity of CO_2 dissociation curve and alveoli CO_2 removal and the lack of a ceiling effect, only marked/extreme increases in Vd/Vt—often to values above 60 percent—will in themselves effect the development of hypercapnia. Such extreme values of Vd/Vt are usually only evident in patients with severe levels of chronic obstructive pulmonary disease (COPD) (associated with FEV1 values less than 30% predicted) and/or severe acute lung injury as occurs during disease processes that cause acute respiratory distress syndrome (ARDS).

Conversely, reductions in V̇e seem to require less-dramatic effects or reductions to lead to the development of hypercapnia from this mechanism alone, realizing that there are two primary mechanisms whereby decreases in V̇e can occur: first, as a consequence of reduced CNS respiratory drive, as commonly occurs in sedative drug overdoses or obesity hypoventilation syndromes; and second, disease states associated with reduced or ineffective neuromuscular effector function involving either decreased CNS transmission through the spinal cord to the phrenic nerve to the diaphragm, direct diaphragmatic muscle disease/dysfunction, or reduced chest-wall movement/expansion. The first mechanism of reduced V̇e is often referred to as patients who "won't breathe," and the second mechanism refers to patients who "can't breathe" because of abnormalities in neuromuscular function and/or chest-wall mechanics (Fahey 1983).

Another important clinical cause of hypercapnia that must be recognized and appropriately treated as a medical or surgical emergency is upper-airway obstruction. The unique physiological principles of the upper airway and trachea render these anatomic areas relatively clinically silent until severe reductions in luminal diameter occur (approximately 1 cm in adults). However, once the upper airway is compromised to this degree, even minor worsening of that obstruction can result in abrupt fatal asphyxia.

References

Berger, A. J. 1988. "Control of Breathing." In *Textbook of Respiratory Medicine*, edited by J. F. Murray and J. A. Nadel. Philadelphia: W. B. Saunders Company. 149–166.

Fahey, P. J., and R. W. Hyde. 1983. "Won't Breathe vs. Can't Breathe." *Chest* 84 (1): 19–25.

Holets, S., and R. D. Hubmayr. 2006. "Setting the Ventilator." In *Principles and Practice of Mechanical Ventilation*, edited by M. J. Tobin. New York: McGraw-Hill, Medical Publishing Division. 163–182.

West, J. B. 1988. "Ventilation, Blood Flow, and Gas Exchange." In *Textbook of Respiratory Medicine*, edited by J. F. Murray and J. A. Nadel. Philadelphia: W. B. Saunders Company. 47–84.

CHAPTER 5

Hypoxemia

• • •

MOST PULMONARY PHYSIOLOGY TEXTBOOKS LIST the following five main causes of hypoxemia: (a) reduced inspired oxygen concentration, (b) hypoventilation, (c) abnormal diffusion, (d) anatomic right to left shunt, and (e) ventilation/perfusion (V/Q) abnormalities or V/Q mismatch. However, in critically ill patients, by far the most common mechanism of hypoxemia is abnormalities in V/Q relationship dominated by lung units with V/Q approaching zero; note that a V/Q = 0 represents a pure anatomic shunt, and a V/Q = 1 represents the "ideal" relationship for optimal gas exchange. This common mechanism of hypoxemia is often referred to as "venous admixture" ($\dot{Q}s/\dot{Q}t$) and is defined as the proportion of mixed venous blood that does not become fully oxygenated as it traverses the pulmonary capillaries and does not equilibrate completely with alveolar gas (usually documented by 0 < V/Q < 1).

Reductions in V/Q producing shuntlike physiology can result from either decreases in the numerator relative to the denominator and/or increases in the denominator relative to the numerator. In either circumstance, capillary blood flow exceeds regional alveolar ventilation. In situations where V/Q ratios have actually been measured using the multiple inert gas elimination technique (MIGET), in general, for various disease states associated with hypoxemia, both venous admixture and true shunt have been demonstrated to some degree.

In nondiseased, healthy individuals, a small degree of pure anatomic shunt (approximately 2–3% of the cardiac output) exists normally. This "normal" shunt volume is caused by (a) bronchial vein blood flow entering the pulmonary veins and (b) thebesian veins of the myocardium emptying directly into the left ventricular cavity without prior mixing with alveolar gas.

In healthy subjects, the range of V/Q dispersion ratios is quite small; more than 95 percent of both ventilation and perfusion is limited to V/Q ratios between 0.3 and 2.1 (Wagner 1974; Laghi 2006). This degree of dispersion increases with age. With pulmonary disease, the V/Q ratio can widen from zero (pure shunt) to infinity (pure dead space). These varying ranges of V/Q ratio dispersion do not refer to the lung unit as a whole; V/Q inequality refers to regional mismatch of ventilation and perfusion (West 1977; Laghi 2006, Figure 5-9).

Compensatory mechanisms tend to minimize effects of abnormal V/Q ratios. The low PaO_2 associated with low V/Q ratios less than 1.0 causes local hypoxic pulmonary vasoconstriction as a compensatory response to improve V/Q ratios, but this compensation remains only partial. However, the greater the magnitude of true shunt, the lower the ability of increased ventilation or even increased inspired fractional concentration of oxygen (FiO_2) to compensate or correct the hypoxemia. In fact, increases in FiO_2 effect little improvement in PaO_2 when the absolute shunt fractions exceed 25 percent of the cardiac output (West 1977; Laghi 2006, Figure 5-11 and Figure 5-8).

In clinical situations of increased dead-space fraction (Vd/Vt), the increased $PaCO_2$ and, to a lesser extent, decreased PaO_2 stimulate central and peripheral chemoreceptors and lead to increased minute ventilation ($\dot{V}e$). In patients without a significant reduction or impairment in ventilator capacity, the increased $\dot{V}e$ is sufficient to bring $PaCO_2$ back to near-normal values, although this increased $\dot{V}e$ has only minimal effects to correct the fall in PaO_2. The different responses of PaO_2 and $PaCO_2$ to increasing levels of ventilation result from the different shapes of the oxygen-hemoglobin (O_2-Hgb) and CO_2 dissociation curves. The O_2-Hgb dissociation curve is flat in the normal range (PaO_2 60 – 100 mmHg), and thus any increase in $\dot{V}e$ or $\dot{V}A$ only benefits lung units on the lower portions of this curve with moderately low V/Q ratios and with little to no effect upon increasing PaO_2 for units in the high normal range. Lung units positioned at the upper portion of the O_2-Hgb dissociation curve (high V/Q ratios) develop minor increases in PaO_2 in the effluent blood; thus, with increased V˙e, mixed PaO_2 rises only moderately, and some degree of hypoxemia always remains. By contrast, the CO_2 dissociation curve is almost linear throughout the normal physiological range, and thus any increases in V˙e or VA immediately raises the CO_2 output from all alveolar units with both high and low V/Q ratios. Similarly, increases in overall ventilation can have a powerful effect upon both PaO_2 and $PaCO_2$ when V/Q dispersion is small. However, with increasing degrees/magnitude of V/Q dispersion, fewer and fewer effects upon PaO_2 and $PaCO_2$ are evident upon increased ventilation. In fact, at extreme degrees of V/Q dispersion, increased ventilation has minimal to no effect upon PaO_2 (West 1977; Laghi 2006, Figure 5-9).

In summary, abnormal V/Q ratios and abnormal V/Q distributions generally do not cause increases in $PaCO_2$ as long as the patient is able to appropriately increase minute ventilation of significant magnitude. However, in relation to PaO_2, similar increases in minute ventilation have effects upon increases in PaO_2 only when V/Q inequality dispersion is relatively normal, but as V/Q inequality dispersion widens, any increase in V˙e is unable to effect any sustained increase to improve PaO_2.

From a lung physiological perspective, most clinical causes of hypoxemia result from individual alveolar units with low V/Q relationships less than the idealized value of 1 and actually approaching 0 (i.e., intrapulmonary alveolar shunts, often referred to as "venous admixture"). Pure anatomic shunts, which represent direct anatomic connections from the venous to the arterial circulation, with V/Q = 0, represent areas of the lung that receive no ventilation but remain perfused, thus not allowing the venous, deoxygenated blood to ever be exposed to the high O_2 content of alveolar gas and thus pass directly through the lungs with end capillary O_2 content and saturation, exactly the same as mixed venous (MVO_2) measurements (under nondisease conditions, MVO_2 = 40 mmHg [75% saturation]).

Although the efficiency of oxygen uptake from the alveoli into capillary blood is quite good, and, under healthy conditions, full equilibration to 100 percent saturation occurs within the first 25 percent of transport time into the alveoli (25 msec), the fact that the saturability of oxygen bound to hemoglobin has peaked at a value of 100 percent is important in dramatically increasing the O_2 carrying capacity and O_2 content of arterial blood being delivered to tissues; however, from the lung perspective, this ceiling effect renders the lung itself vulnerable to derangements in oxygen uptake and does not allow compensatory nondiseased alveoli to make up for the reduced oxygen saturations entering the left atrium from diseased alveoli and thus emerging into the systemic circulation with oxygen saturations less than 100 percent. Thus, in contrast to CO_2 balance, where major changes in Vd/Vt must occur to affect hypercapnia, in relation to PaO_2, relatively minor changes can at times cause severe and noncorrectable levels of hypoxemia not improved by the simple addition of supplemental oxygen.

Examples of this mechanism of hypoxemia resultant from abnormal venous admixture include patients with acute bacterial pneumonia whereby the large areas of airway and parenchymal consolidation fail to ventilate normally, although—if the associated pulmonary circulation were able to adapt exactly through hypoxic vasoconstriction to precisely reduce the amount of perfusion to that focal area to amount reduction in ventilation—then indeed V/Q would be preserved and normal oxygenation preserved. However, given the high-output cardiac state associated with an acute systemic infectious process and, even more importantly, the paralysis of hypoxic vasoconstriction in the area of acute airway/parenchyma inflammation, infection, and consolidation, large volumes of pulmonary arterial blood flow are shunted through the diseased area in absence of exposure to oxygenated alveoli, and hypoxemia ensues.

Another instructive example of this mechanism of hypoxemia is evident in cases of acute pulmonary embolism. Simplistically, theorize that thrombotic emboli occludes 25 percent of the pulmonary circulation; then indeed, per that specific localized regional area, because of a decrease in the V/Q denominator, V/Q would increase and manifest as increased dead space, which indeed does occur. However, the full pre-event cardiac output still needs to be maintained to perfuse adequately the systemic circulation; and because, at any beat of the heart, the same volume ejected from the left ventricle equals that ejected from right ventricle, these areas with preserved/normal ventilation and nonthrombotic/embolic occlusion now become overperfused (because of an increase in V/Q denominator) by the volume of blood shunted away from the occluded pulmonary vascular disease, now redistributed to the healthy areas, which then in essence causes a decrease in V/Q (i.e., shuntlike physiology) because of increased $\dot{Q}$ and resultant clinical hypoxemia.

For the intensivist, two additional but infrequently considered mechanisms of hypoxemia merit consideration. First, in acute lung injury of large enough magnitude to severely reduce the pulmonary vascular circulatory volume or surface area, acute marked elevations in right-heart pressures and acute cor pulmonale can develop, which, if significant in magnitude, can actually physiologically induce the opening of the foramen ovale and cause a resultant pure anatomic shunt from right to left. The second mechanism involves disease states associated with severe reductions in systemic perfusion, as occurs in such disease states (either hypovolemic or cardiogenic shock) where systemic capillary-tissue oxygen extraction mechanisms remain intact. Tissue adaptation to reductions in O_2 delivery (DO_2) results in increased compensatory oxygen extraction at the systemic capillary level, but only to a certain limit (maximal increase approximately 75%). This increased tissue O_2 extraction results in reduced levels of venous blood returning to the right atrium from the venous blood exiting highly metabolic tissues so that MVO_2 saturations are commonly less than the normal nondisease, healthy value of 40 mmHg (75% saturation), often approximating values of 27 mmHg (50% saturation). In situations of overt clinical lung disease in association with existent abnormal increases in absolute shunt or shunt fraction, these reduced values of mixed venous blood oxygenation only serve to reduce to an even greater extent the already decreased oxygen contents entering the left side of the heart (West 1977; West 1991, Figure 5).

REFERENCES

Laghi, F., and M. J. Tobin. 2006. "Indications for Mechanical Ventilation." In *Principles and Practice of Mechanical Ventilation*, edited by M. J. Tobin. New York: McGraw-Hill, Medical Publishing Division. 129–160.

Wagner, P. D., R. B. Laravuso, R. R. Uhl, and J. B. West. 1974. "Continuous Distributions of Ventilation Perfusion Ratios in Normal Subjects Breathing Air and 100% O_2." *Journal of Clinical Investigation* 54: 54–68.

West, J. B. 1977. "State of the Art: Ventilation Perfusion Relationships." *American Review of Respiratory Disease* 116: 919–943.

West, J. B., and P. D. Wagner. 1991. "Ventilation Perfusion Relationships." In *The Lung Scientific Foundations*, edited by R. G. Crystal. New York: Raven Press. 1289–1305.

CHAPTER 6

The Upper Airway

• • •

THE UPPER AIRWAY IS DEFINED as the part of the conducting airway between the nose and the main carina located at the end of the distal trachea (Braman 1998). The upper airway includes the nasal and oral cavities, pharynx, larynx, and trachea. It must be noted that although the nose and oral cavity have redundant and parallel pathways for airway flow, the remainder of the upper-airway structures consist of a single-orifice, tubular structure whose complete obstruction will result in immediate asphyxia. The upper airways make a large, variable contribution to total airway resistance—as much as 50 percent in normal subjects during mouth breathing but only about 20 percent in subjects with diseases of the small peripheral airways causing chronic airflow limitation, because in the presence of diffuse small airway disease, the absolute values of airway resistance (Raw) of the lower airways increase more than those of the upper airways (Hyatt 1961). Although the patency of the upper airways is a complex interaction of neuromuscular control, virtually for all critical-care diseases, the bulk of acute upper-airway obstruction (UAO), both partial and complete, results from anatomic mass occlusion/obstruction. There are a variety of clinical disorders that can cause UAO, including infections, trauma, anaphylaxis, congenital defects, vascular malformations, and both benign and malignant masses. In relation to critical-care medicine, postintubation endotracheal tube-related laryngeal and tracheal complications probably represent the most commonly experienced acute cause of UAO.

In relation to any specific disease process or etiology, the importance of timely and effective management lies not only with an accurate diagnosis but also with an accurate assessment of time frame in relation to the onset, development, and progression of UAO. Some diseases, such as acute anaphylaxis, can cause immediate suffocation and death from massive tissue swelling and edema. Others, such as tracheal tumors or papillomatosis, are more indolent, long-term developing disease processes, but they can eventually progress to the same level of severity. In addition, dependent upon specific anatomic location, UAO may be variable, meaning that the degree and magnitude of obstructions varies with the specific phases of respiration. Structures located above the thoracic inlet constitute the extrathoracic airway, and the portion below the thoracic inlet make up the intrathoracic upper airway (Braman 1998). In variable UAO, forces and pressures, both internal and external to the particular anatomically located tubular structure (i.e., transluminal pressure gradients), will have different respiratory-phase flow changes in relation to either the presence or absence of obstruction and its severity. In general, in cases of variable extrathoracic obstruction, increased Raw is manifest predominantly on inspiration resultant from the Bernoulli effect, with expiratory flow being near normal. In relation to variable intrathoracic obstruction, airway lumina dilate on inspiration but occlude on expiration because expiratory-phase transmural airway pressure favors occlusion and collapse. In cases of fixed UAO, flow is fixed or constant during all phases of respiration without variability between inspiration or expiration (Miller 1973).

However, regardless of the respiratory phase of UAO, the basic physiological principles are the same: to develop symptoms or signs of UAO, the degree or magnitude of airway occlusion must be relatively severe. This is why it is critically important to understand that any symptom related to UAO (especially dyspnea) and, in particular, any degree, even very minor, of documented hypercapnia represent a medical/surgical emergency (Al-Qadi 2013).

Multiple studies have demonstrated that the normal transverse diameter of the adult trachea is approximately 13–25 mm for males and approximately 10–23 mm in females, with an overall mean value of 18.4 mm. The anterioposterior diameter approximates 15–28 mm (20.1) (Brown 1983; Breatnach 1984; Holbert 1995). In relation to UAO physiology, in general, dyspnea on exertion will not be evident until the airway lumen is reduced approximately 75–80 percent from its normal diameter to absolute measurement of approximately 8 mm, in comparison to the usual trachea diameter, which can be as large as 25 mm (Ernst 2004; Brouns 2007). Dyspnea at rest and imminent suffocation will then occur at a relatively trivial further reduction to a value of 5 mm in diameter (Braman 1998; Ernst 2004).

The central importance of the airway/tube radius in determining driving airway pressure and the critical determinant of airway/tubular resistance is apparent from the relationship based upon Poiseulle's equation noting that if airway/tube radius is halved, then the pressure gradient required to maintain a given flow must be increased sixteenfold ([R = (8/Π) × (L/r^4) × nu], where R = resistance; L = length; r = radius; nu = viscosity). As relates to the physiology and also pathophysiology of any flow through any tubular structures, especially in relation to clinical cases of UAO, the determinants of Raw include not only the anatomic characteristics of the tube but also the flow rate being generated by respiratory muscular effort or mechanical ventilation (van Noord 1987). Studies have identified the importance of both factors in contributing to increases inspiratory Raw for patients with variety of causes of anatomic UAO. Thus, for similar degrees of anatomic occlusion, the higher the flow rate, the greater the Raw (Brouns 2007, Figure 5), and thus the greater the resultant spontaneous or mechanical pressure work to maintain adequate ventilation and gas exchange. This principle is especially important in relation to increased Raw and increased WOB related to high inspiratory flow rates in patients intubated with endotracheal tubes of less than 6 mm in internal diameter, whereby flow becomes a significant factor contributing to the resistive component of the increased work of breathing (WOB) (Wright 1989, Figures 3, 4, 5, 6).

Absolute measurements of Raw and respiratory system resistance (Rrs) (cmH$_2$O/L/sec) obtained from three groups of patients with (a) variable extrathoracic obstruction, (b) fixed UAO, or (c) variable intrathoracic obstruction and their dependence upon flow rates and phase of respiration is evident in the accompanying Table 6.1 (Miller 1973; van Noord 1987).

Table 6.1 Measurements of Airway Resistance (Raw) and Respiratory System Resistance (Rrs) Relative to Anatomic Site of Upper-Airway Obstruction and Flow Rate

	Variable-Extrathoracic	Fixed	Variable-Intrathoracic
	cmH$_2$O/L/sec	cmH$_2$O/L/sec	cmH$_2$O/L/sec
Inspiration ($\dot{V}i = 0.5$ L/sec)	1.84 +/− 1.12	3.67 +/− 1.43	2.65–3.26
Inspiration ($\dot{V}i = 1.0$ L/sec)	2.55 +/− 1.63	6.12 +/− 2.96	3.98–5.71
Inspiration (Rrs)	7.6 +/− 0.9	8.1 +/− 1.7	5.6 +/− 1.5
Expiration (Rrs)	5.5 +/− 0.6	6.4 +/− 1.2	4.7 +/− 1.1

Other studies have demonstrated even more marked elevations in Raw for seven patients with UAO with values ranging from 4.1 cmH$_2$O/L/sec (469% of predicted normal) to 22.0 cmH$_2$O/L/sec (1,667 % of predicted normal) (Sackner 1972). These measurements represented Raw values five to eighteen times the normal level (Sackner 1972). This same study also allowed the direct correlation of increased Raw with actual intraluminal tracheal diameter: 6 mm, corresponding to Raw 17.7 cmH$_2$O/L/sec; 6–7 mm corresponding to Raw 10.6 cmH$_2$O/L/sec (Sackner 1972).

The magnitude of these elevations in Raw attributed to lesions of the upper airway can actually exceed values observed in patients with asthma or COPD whereby the majority of the increased WOB and increased Raw is attributable to disease of the small peripheral airways (i.e., terminal bronchioles with an internal diameter less than 2 mm). Finally, utilizing invasive bronchoscopic techniques in attempts to localize exact sites of tracheal obstruction with the intent of accurately identifying the exact site stent placement, these same physiological principles were also verified. This study demonstrated that for any significant difference in pressure development measured at the lateral walls at two separate anatomic sites with intent to identify the flow-limiting segment as an indicator of increased resistance, tracheal luminal diameter had to be reduced in magnitude to greater than 60 percent intraluminal narrowing before the flow-limiting segment could be identified/evident with exponential increase in pressure difference with further degrees of worsening UAO (Nishine 2012, Figure 2).

References

Al-Qadi, M. O., A. W. Artenstein, and S. S. Braman. 2013. "The 'Forgotten Zone': Acquired Disorders of the Trachea in Adults." *Respiratory Medicine* 107: 1301–1313.

Braman, S. S., and H. A. Gaissert. 1998. "Upper Airway Obstruction." In *Fishman's Pulmonary Diseases and Disorders*, edited by A. P. Fishman. New York: McGraw-Hill, Health Professions Division. 781–801.

Breatnach, E., G. C. Abbott, and R. G. Fraser. 1984. "Dimensions of the Normal Human Trachea." *American Journal of Roentgenology* 142: 903–906.

Brouns, M., S. T. Jayaraju, C. Lacor, J. De Mey, M. Noppen, W. Vincken, and S. Verbanck. 2007. "Tracheal Stenosis: A Flow Dynamic Study." *Journal of Applied Physiology* 102: 1178–1184.

Brown, B. M., A. K. Oshita, and R. A. Castellino. 1983. "CT Assessment of the Adult Extrathoracic Trachea." *Journal of Computerized Assisted Tomography* 7 (3): 415–418.

Ernst, A., D. Feller-Kopman, H. D. Becker, and A. C. Mehta. 2004. "Central Airway Obstruction." *American Journal of Respiratory and Critical Care Medicine* 169: 1278–1297.

Holbert, J. M., and D. C. Strollo. 1995. "Imaging of the Normal Trachea." *Journal of Thoracic Imaging* 10: 171–179.

Hyatt, R. E., and R. E. Wilcox. 1961. "Extrathoracic Airway Resistance in Man." *Journal of Applied Physiology* 16: 326–330.

Miller, R. D., and R. E. Hyatt. 1973. "Evaluation of Obstructing Lesions of the Trachea and Larynx by Flow-Volume Loops." *American Review of Respiratory Disease* 108: 475–481.

Nishine, H., T. Hiramoto, H. Kida, S. Matsuoka, M. Mineshita, N. Kurimoto, and T. Miyazawa. 2012. "Assessing the Site of Maximal Obstruction in the Trachea Using Lateral Pressure Measurement during Bronchoscopy." *American Journal of Respiratory and Critical Care Medicine* 185 (1): 24–33.

Sackner, M. A. 1972. "Physiologic Features of Upper Airway Obstruction." *Chest* 62 (4): 414–417.

Van Noord, J. A., W. Wellens, I. Clarysse, M. Cauberghs, K. P. Van de Woestijne, and M. Demedts. 1987. "Total Respiratory Resistance and Reactance in Patients with Upper Airway Obstruction." *Chest* 92: 475–480.

Wright, P. E., J. J. Marini, G. R. Bernard. 1989. "In Vitro vs. In Vivo Comparison of Endotracheal Tube Airflow Resistance." *American Review of Respiratory Disease* 140: 10–16.

CHAPTER 7

Mechanics

• • •

Transpulmonary Pressure and Static Pressure/Volume Relationship

Ventilation, which includes lung inflation and chest-wall expansion, requires muscular effort/work in spontaneously breathing individuals and mechanical ventilator work for intubated patients requiring invasive mechanical support. This concept of "work" is usually referenced in relation to pressure changes required to achieve and sustain ventilation. In the case of the lung, the elastic work of breathing (WOB) is required to overcome the natural tendency of the lung to recoil to its collapsed position (which, in the absence of the intact chest wall, will be a volume less than functional residual capacity [FRC]), whereas the nonelastic work is done to overcome both the resistances to airflow and the viscous resistances of the lung tissue to deformation. This WOB can, under healthy conditions, be partitioned into (a) 63.3 percent to overcome the elastic work of inspiration, (b) 28.5 percent to overcome the resistive component of the work of inspiration, and (c) 8.2 percent to overcome the forces of tissue deformation during inspiration (Otis 1950). The elastic behavior of the lung depends on two factors: the physical properties of the lung tissue and the surface tension of the film lining the air-alveolar (gas-liquid) interface. The tissue components contributing to lung elasticity are (a) pleura, (b) intralobular septa, (c) peripheral airways, (d) smooth muscle tone, and (e) tissues of the alveolar wall composed predominately of collagen and elastin.

The fibrous skeleton of the lung is the structure that bears the mechanical forces of stress. This skeleton consists of two fiber systems: an axial system, which is anchored to the hilum and runs along the branching airways down to the alveolar ducts, and a peripheral system, which is anchored to the visceral pleura that extend centripetally down into the lung to the acini. The two systems are linked at the level of the alveolus and form a continuous structure. The anatomic units of this system are extensible elastin and inextensible collagen, which is folded/pleated in the lung resting position. Elastic fibers have low tensile strength but can be stretched to more than twice their resting length. Collagen fibers have high tensile strength and act to limit expansion at high lung volumes. The limits of distention are dictated by the inextensible collagen fibers, which act as the stop-length system. When the collagen fibers are fully unfolded, the lungs reach their maximal volume, and further elongation is prevented. The lung cells themselves do not bear force but are anchored to this fibrous skeleton and must accommodate their shape when the framework is distended. This is true for the whole lung as well as for each lung region, which has its own total "regional" maximal capacity.

The movement of air into the lung during inspiration requires the creation of pressure gradients to effect flow and then volume expansion. From a purely mechanical work perspective, the process of breathing can simplistically be viewed in terms of three variables: pressure, flow, and volume—which, by the way, are exactly the three physiological parameters displayed visually on most modern mechanical ventilators. The medical literature uses multiple and at times different phrases and terminologies to reflect the various pressure changes requisite for ventilation. For understanding rather than focus upon the exact wording or terms, emphasis should be placed upon comprehending their concepts.

Transpulmonary pressure (Ptp) represents the total pressure gradient generated across the lung during various phases on inspiratory muscle effort when breathing spontaneously or through mechanical ventilator effort when receiving invasive ventilation. The transpulmonary pressure is also frequently referred to as the "trans-lung" pressure (Truwit and Marini 1988). Ptp is defined as the pressure difference between Pao (airway opening pressure) or Pm (mouth pressure) and pleural pressure (Ppl). Ptp is the sum of three pressure elements: (a) Pel (elastic distending pressure), (b) Pfr (flow resistance pressure), and (c) Pin (pressure to overcome inertia). Ptp can be further divided into subcomponents: Ptp = (Pao – Palv) + (Palv – Ppl) = Pao – Ppl. Flow through the airways is generated by the transairway pressure (i.e., Pao – Palv), which is the pressure gradient required to overcome the resistance to flow of the tracheobronchial tree. Expansion of the elastic compartment is generated by the transthoracic pressure (i.e., Palv – Ppl). Although it is convenient to think of the pleural pressure as a single value, marked heterogeneity exists in relation to position, gravity, body habitus, and disease—nonetheless, thinking of pleural pressure as a single value has practical significance. Under conditions of no flow, Palv = Pao, and thus transpulmonary pressure becomes Palv – Ppl, which represents the forces necessary to overcome only the distending or elastic (nonresistive) components of ventilation (Truwit and Marini 1988, Figure 1; Grippi 1998, Figure 36-7; Fishman 1998, Appendix C-4; Warner 2000, Figure 1; Chatburn 2006, Figure 2-1).

However, during either spontaneous breathing or mechanical ventilation, the process of respiration requires *both* the inflation of the lung and also the expansion of the chest wall. Thus, in addition, a third component of WOB must be performed to overcome compliance forces of the chest wall, whose pressure gradient represents the difference between Ppl and Patm (i.e., Ppl – Patm). Thus the distending pressure for the elastic work of the entire respiratory system represents the sum of these two pressure gradients: Presp = (Palv – P pl) + (Ppl – Patm) = Palv – Patm. Thus, summing all of the critical components (elastic and nonelastic) during any inspiratory effort represents the sums of (Pao – Palv) + (Palv – Ppl) + (Ppl – Patm) = Pao – Patm. For critically ill patients receiving invasive positive-pressure ventilation, the transrespiratory pressure (pressure at the airway opening minus pressure on the body surface) is the total pressure required to generate inspiration (Truwit and Marini 1988).

Air moves in and out of the lungs whenever the sum of pressures developed by passive recoil of the respiratory system and by the respiratory muscles (or mechanical ventilation) is other than zero. During spontaneous breathing, the actions of the inspiratory muscles cause an increase in the outward recoil of the chest wall; as a result, pleural pressure becomes reduced relative to atmospheric pressure (i.e., subatmospheric). This pressure change is transmitted to the interior of the lungs, so alveolar pressure also becomes subatmospheric—hence the term "negative-pressure ventilation." In contrast, during mechanical ventilation with a positive-pressure breathing machine, a supra-atmospheric pressure applied at the inlet of the airways creates the necessary pressure gradient between the airway opening and alveoli to achieve volume expansion and subsequent ventilation.

If the integrity of the lung and chest wall is breached, the natural physiological tendency of the lung as an individual unit is to collapse inward and the chest wall as an individual unit to expand outward. However, when functioning as a single, intact, synchronous system, the tendency for the lungs to deflate inwardly is counterbalanced by the outwardly directed elastic recoil of the chest wall. When at rest in the absence of any respiratory muscle activity, these opposing forces generate a subatmospheric pleural pressure approximately –5 cmH_2O and keep the lungs in an inflated state with a volume of gas exactly equal to functional residual capacity (FRC). Note that even in the "resting" state, in the absence of muscular activity at end expiration, the volume of retained gas within the lungs and thorax in association with appreciable concentrations or stores of oxygen is significant, approximately 2–3 L in volume and 400–600 mL in O_2 reservoir in spontaneously breathing subjects in the absence of supplemental oxygen (Schlobohm 1981).

Remarkably, under healthy conditions, the respiratory system is designed to utilize muscular effort only during inspiration but to then harness that stored energy to accomplish the full task of breathing; that is, the requisite expiratory phase of ventilation. Expiration is usually and predominately a passive physiological process in the absence of expiratory muscle activation. As previously noted, passive expiratory flow is generated by the energy stored in the elastic components of the lung and chest wall during inspiration. Note that as the lung and chest wall expand in association with positive values for Ptp, these stored forces then represent accumulated recoil pressure directing flow outward during expiration. Work done during inspiration is stored in the elastic structures of the respiratory system and is then available as the power supply to passive expiration. As lung volume increases, the total respiratory system recoil pressure becomes positive because of two factors: the increased inward elastic recoil of the lung and the decreased outward elastic recoil of the chest wall.

The mechanical properties of the respiratory system are best depicted by plotting transpulmonary pressure (Ptp) on the horizontal axis and volume on the vertical axis. The pressure-volume (P-V) characteristics of the elastic component of the WOB can then be expressed in one of three configurations: (a) the lung itself, (b) the chest wall itself, or (c) the summation of lung + chest wall. Ptp is often expressed either in reference to resting pressure (+ or − referenced to zero) or in absolute values of intrapleural pressure. Volume is often expressed in relation to resting lung volume at FRC and expressed as percent of total lung capacity (TLC). Characteristics of this pressure-volume (P-V) relationship in healthy, nondiseased states are well characterized and demonstrated in accompanying references/citations.

Notice also that the P-V relationship of the total respiratory system represents the summation of these separate P-V relationships and that for each individual component to increase or expand upon inspiration, the similar forces of resistance, compliance, and inertia must be overcome. Under static (inspiratory-hold) conditions, in the absence of flow, the static P-V curve depicts only the components of the elastic WOB (i.e., lung compliance or lung elastance). It is sometimes convenient to think of the static P-V curve not as the pressure needed to inflate the lungs and expand the chest wall but rather as the distending pressures required to *keep* the lungs inflated and the chest wall expanded.

During the majority of inspiration at lung volumes above FRC (i.e., the resting volume of the lungs and thorax), the outward recoil of the chest wall actually assists/augments the physiological process of lung expansion, and thus its outwardly directed recoil pressure is subtracted from the remainder of the WOB, which, in effect, serves to reduce Ptp for the majority of lung volume expansion. At lung volumes above FRC, the elastic recoil of the lung compresses alveolar gas, raising Palv > Pb or P mouth, thus assisting expiration passively. At lung volumes below FRC, the relaxation pressure measured at the mouth is negative because the outward recoil of the chest wall is now greater than the reduced inward recoil of the lungs, thus assisting inspiration passively. However, at high lung volumes, in the latter 20 percent of P-V curve expansion toward TLC, at the point where the chest-wall P-V curve crosses the vertical axis at zero Ptp, the chest wall becomes overexpanded, and now active muscle pressure must be generated to actually overcome this inward chest-wall recoil force, and thus the total pressure of respiration is now added to the Ptp, now requiring greater degrees of pressure gradient generation to maintain lung expansion at the upper limits of the P-V curve. Again, remember that the extra pressure to attain inspiration then becomes stored energy or pressure to passively assist expiration. In summary, at thoracic volumes below 70 percent TLC, the chest wall's elastic recoil is outward, and at volumes above 70 percent TLC, the chest wall's recoil pressure is inward (Collett 1988, Figure 5-30).

Notice (especially in relation to the lung-specific P-V curve/characteristics) the multiple phase transitions of this relationship, including a relatively flat portion/phase at the beginning of inspiratory effort whereby little effective lung volume expansion occurs early, but then a remarkable transition into a steep, exponentially increasing phase whereby little changes in pressure effect large increments in volume and finally a return to a flat curve, again demonstrating the fixed and limited expansion capacity of the static lung. Also evident upon review of the static P-V curve is the importance of the maintenance of FRC and prevention of a "gasless" lung that ideally positions the resting lung volumes at the relatively steep portion of this P-V curve, thus allowing for much greater changes in volume (ΔV) for any given change in pressure (ΔP) (Weinberger 1998, Figure 250-3; West 2005; Figure 7-11). In addition, this "gasless" lung, as previously noted, deprives the respiratory system of a reservoir of alveolar O_2 for continuous uptake at the alveolar capillary level even at times of inactive inspiration.

Lung/Chest Wall Compliance and Elastance

The elastic properties of the respiratory system in both health and disease are often inferred from measurements of respiratory systems compliance or its inverse elastance. Compliance is measured under static no-flow conditions and is calculated as change in lung volume for a given change in distending pressure ($\Delta V/\Delta P$). Sometimes, for ease of understanding, the term "elastance" (cmH_2O/L), which is the reciprocal of "compliance" (L/cmH_2O), is also used to describe these various pressure differences. This term is more analogous in terminology to the concept of airway resistance (Raw) and better reflects the importance of pressure change necessary to effect volume expansion ($\Delta P/\Delta V$, expressed in units cmH_2O/L), rather than vice versa as compliance depicts ($\Delta V/\Delta P$, expressed in unit L/cmH_2O). Elastance can be measured as either *static* elastance by plotting data at times without airflow during an interrupted inflation or deflation or as *dynamic* elastance by plotting data at end-expiration and end-inspiration instants at zero flow. Thus, static and dynamic elastance values differ on the basis of volume history. Normal values for chest wall and lung dynamic elastance approximate 5 cmH_2O/L each, resulting in measurements of the total summed/added respiratory system elastance, usually measuring 10 cmH_2O/L (Katz 1981; Loring 2009). Measurements of elastance reflect a more linear distribution of elastic recoil when examining characteristics of the lung and chest wall, as these components are additive (Katz 1981). In addition, in disease states associated with increased elastic recoil of either the lung, chest wall, or both, this change will be reflected by a larger increase in elastance rather than a decrease in measurement of compliance.

In addition, the lungs and chest wall behave as elements coupled in series. Thus, to measure the combined compliance of both components (Clung + Ccw) and, in effect, then calculate the compliance of the total respiratory system (Ctotal, rs), their reciprocals are added: 1/Ctotal, rs = 1/Clung + 1/Ccw (Sharp 1991).

Given the dynamic characteristics of the lung and the entire respiratory system, lung compliance is not constant; it changes with lung volume, reflecting the curvilinear nature of the P-V curve. Numerically, total thoracic compliance is calculated from the relationship between these two capacitance elements (lung and chest wall) coupled in series by the equation 1/Ctotal = 1/Clung + 1/C chest wall (Truwit and Marini 1988; Ward 1994). During spontaneous breathing in normal, healthy individuals, the compliance of the normal chest wall and normal lung are each approximately 200 mL/cmH_2O; thus, the expected/calculated total respiratory system compliance would be 100 mL/cm-H_2O (Sharp 1964; Truwit and Marini 1988). Diseases of the lung itself, such as pneumonia, lung fibrosis, or acute respiratory distress syndrome (ARDS), will result in increased lung elastance (Elung) or increased lung stiffness or, inversely, decreased lung compliance (Clung) with concomitant increased work of breathing (WOB) for the entire respiratory system. Abnormalities in chest-wall compliance (Ccw) can occur in relation to a number of disease processes that will also proportionally increase the overall respiratory system WOB and include kyphosoliosis; ankylosing spondylitis; chest-wall deformities such as flail chest, pectus carinatum, and pectus excavatum; and—probably of greatest significance to the critical-care physician—obesity.

However, as shown in the accompanying table, even in the absence of intrinsic lung disease, in critically ill supine patients on mechanical ventilation also receiving sedation and with minimal respiratory muscle activity, these same measurements of compliance, when measured and calculated, are not of the same magnitude or values as the awake, healthy, upright, spontaneously breathing volunteer subjects;

other factors such as the inelasticity and resistance of the endotracheal tube and the resistance and compliance factors of the ventilator equipment itself are also components contributing to the overall decreases in compliance measurements for critically ill patients compared to healthy, nondiseased volunteers. Yet the same physiological principles apply, again noting the dependence of lung compliance upon lung volumes and the curvilinear nature of the P-V curve. Some representative values of healthy subjects and a variety of ICU critically ill patients receiving invasive mechanical ventilation are provided in the accompanying Tables 7.1, 7.2, and 7.3 (C = compliance [mL/cmH$_2$O]; E = elastance [cm H$_2$O/L]).

Table 7.1: Elastic Respiratory Mechanics (Compliance and Elastance) in Health and Disease. (Grimby 1975)

	Ctot[mL/cmH$_2$O]	Clung[mL/cmH$_2$O]	Ccw[mL/cmH$_2$O]
Patients "free from respiratory disease"	44.8 ± 4.4 (Vt = 386 mL +/− 29)	74.1 ± 15.0	108.6 ± 38.8
	56.2 ± 6.3 (Vt = 722 mL +/− 67)	94.3 ± 20.4	152.3 ± 44.0
	56.5 ± 5.7 (Vt = 1126 mL +/− 187)	88.7 ± 16.9	167.6 ± 43.9

Table 7.2: Elastic Respiratory Mechanics (Compliance and Elastance) in Health and Disease (C = compliance [mL/cmH$_2$O]; E = elastance [cm H$_2$O/L]). (Katz 1981)

	Ctot	Clung	Ccw	Etot	Elung	Ecw
Critically ill population	36	54	106	28 ± 3	19 ± 2	9.4 ± 1

Table 7.3: Elastic Respiratory Mechanics (Compliance and Elastance) in Health and Disease. (Chiumello 2008) (ARDS = acute respiratory distress syndrome/ALI = acute lung injury)

	Ctot (mL/cmH$_2$O)	Etot (cmH$_2$O/L)
Surgical Controls	56 ± 16	19 ± 6
Medical Controls	45 ± 11	24 ± 6
ARDS	42 ± 14	26 ± 8
ALI	47 ± 18	24 ± 9

Also refer to detailed Figure 7 in Rittayamai et al. (2015), "Pressure-Controlled vs. Volume-Controlled Ventilation in Acute Respiratory Failure: A Physiology-Based Narrative and Systematic Review" (in *Chest* 148 [2]: 340–355).

The magnitude of the component of the pressure (and subsequent work) required to overcome the various resistive (nonelastic) and capacitance (elastic) elements of ventilation and the WOB can be somewhat estimated from review of the pressure-volume characteristics of the mechanical ventilator. The total or peak airway pressure (Ppeak) recorded from the mechanical ventilator manometer or pressure gauge indicator is the measurement of force necessary to overcome both compliance and resistive work to affect an adequate lung expansion for gas exchange. If, after the completion of a full inspiratory effort, flow is stopped by inducing an inspiratory pause or hold, then in essence, the pressure remaining in the ventilator circuit is simply the pressure required to maintain the lung in a constant nonflow distended inflation. When the volume of gas in the lungs and airways is held constant so that flow and volume acceleration are zero, all the pressure readings related to flow resistance and inertia are also zero. This rapid airway occlusion at the end of a passive inspiratory phase of ventilation procedure produces an *immediate* drop in both airway pressure (Paw) and transpulmonary pressure (Ptp) from a peak pressure (Ppeak) to a lower initial value (Pinit) *followed* by a *gradual* decrease in pressure until plateau (Pplat) pressure is achieved after three to five seconds of occlusion (Fernandez-Perez 2006; Singer 2009). Under these no-flow conditions, the pressure manometer or pressure monitor will drop, and the difference between the peak airway pressure (Ppeak) and this static pressure, called the plateau pressure (Pplat), represents the pressure or forces necessary to generate flow in the airway tubular branching system and thus represents the resistive component of WOB. The remaining component of the total WOB represents the forces or pressure necessary to overcome the compliance characteristics of the lung—that is, the pressure difference between Pplat and pressure at end expiration (Pend-expiration) (Truwit and Marini 1988; Tobin 1988, Figure 6; Tobin 1990, Figure 3; Ward 1994, Figure 4-43; Jubran 1995; Jubran 1996, Figure 9; Dhand 1995, Figure 1; Gattinoni 2006; Singer 2009; Hess 2014, Figure 1).

Using this technique, both the compliance component and resistive component of the WOB can also be estimated from review of the pressure characteristics of the mechanical ventilator circuitry. Under static conditions at zero airflow, the actual compliance can then be calculated or, more commonly, inferred by calculating the distending pressure measured as the difference from where the breath starts (end expiration) to plateau pressure value (i.e., Crs, total = Vt/[Pplateau – Pend-expiration]) in units mL/cmH$_2$O (Jubran 1996). If patients are receiving positive end-expiratory pressure (PEEP) as a component of their mechanical ventilation strategy, then Pend -expiratory = PEEP. Recently, Pplateau has become a major focus of ventilatory strategies for ARDS with strong current recommendations with supportive clinical outcome data validating the concept of keeping this value below 30 cmH$_2$O as improving both survival and ventilator-free days in this population of critically ill high-mortality patients. In addition, Raw can be estimated in a similar manner by measuring the pressure drop (i.e., difference) between Ppk and Pplat divided by the inspiratory flow ([Ppk – Pplat]/V̇i), expressed as cm H$_2$O/L/sec (Singer 2009; Gattinoni 2006).

Recent studies have attempted to refine the relationship between tidal volume (Vt), positive end-expiratory pressure (PEEP), and implementation of the lung protection ventilation strategy upon multiple clinical outcomes in critically ill and post-operative patients requiring invasive mechanical ventilation. Two publications analyzing previously reported clinical trials data in patients with ARDS and post-operative patients have shown a relationship between higher levels of a calculated derived value termed "driving pressure" and worse clinical outcomes (Amato 2015; Neto 2016). By definition, driving pressure equals Vt/Crs which in effect is calculated as the difference between the ventilator induced plateau pressure (Pplat) and the level of PEEP (Pplat — PEEP). Specifically, analyses of this retrospective data seemed to indicate that there were thresholds for driving pressure above which there was a relationship between higher driving pressures and mortality in ARDS patients and a composite term of pulmonary complications in post-operative patients. These speculations still require formal confirmation and validation in well-designed prospective and randomized clinical trials but merit comment.

As previously discussed for the normal, nondiseased lung, these same principles apply to diseased lungs also, but obviously as the degree of lung effacement, consolidation, and destruction becomes greater, the compliance portion of the requisite work of breathing in critically ill patients becomes excessive, frequently creating an excessive load that the respiratory muscles cannot overcome, and acute respiratory failure (ARF) ensues. For these reasons, the importance of surfactant in reducing airway surface tension and minimizing the compliance component of the WOB becomes all the more obvious. In fact, ARF of the neonate is a direct consequence of failure of alveolar type II cells to mature to a level that can effect sufficient surfactant production to ease this WOB, and ARF frequently ensues (termed the neonatal respiratory distress syndrome). In fact, exogenous administration of inhaled synthetic surfactant is one of the few FDA-approved drugs for infants and neonates. Even though altered or deficient surfactant production from diseased or necrotic type II pneumocytes is probably also a factor leading to reduced compliance in various adult disease states, including ARDS, for multiple reasons, including chemical composition, method of delivery, and lung deposition, augmentation of surfactant to the alveoli by exogenous administration has proven ineffective in modifying clinical outcomes in clinical cases of ARDS.

AIRWAY RESISTANCE AND THE DYNAMIC PHASE OF BREATHING/RESPIRATION

Acknowledging the previous principles in relation to the static/no-flow characteristics and the elastic properties of the P-V curve of the lung and chest wall, additional pressure generation must be achieved to overcome the nonelastic or resistive forces to effect overall ventilation. Airway resistance (Raw) represents the frictional component of inflation impedance and is defined as the ratio of driving pressure divided by flow and is usually expressed as $cmH_2O/L/sec$. Raw is the work required to overcome the resistive forces of air moving down a branching tubular structure. Under dynamic conditions of flow, the P-V curve changes when airflow is added, both increasing the amount of pressure necessary to effect increases in volume and also the curious development of the process of hysteresis whereby the inflation portion of the curve is markedly different from the deflation portion of the curve when airflow or dynamicity is added. Hysteresis is the failure of a system to follow identical paths of response upon application and withdrawal of a forcing agent. Most of the hysteresis in the air-filled lung is due to surface tension forces. This is because surface tension of the material lining the alveoli is higher during inflation, when the surface film is expanding, than during deflation, when the surface film is being compressed.

Using the same mechanical ventilation occlusion technique, and again noting that the difference between Ppeak and Pplateau represents the mechanical work to overcome Raw in critically ill patients, Raw can actually be estimated by taking that pressure difference and dividing by inspiratory flow ($\dot{V}i$), calculated as Raw = (Ppeak − Pplat)/$\dot{V}i$, expressed as $cmH_2O/L/sec$.

The branching structure of the airways can be grouped as (a) conducting, (b) distributing, and (c) gas exchange. In health, the resistance of the airways below the larynx is dominated by the resistance of the larger, more central airways where flow is turbulent and transitional. As the airways continue to branch distally, the airway diameter narrows, but the surface area increases dramatically. Under healthy, nondisease conditions, the bulk of this Raw is generated by the large airways, with the small airways (defined as terminal bronchioles with an internal diameter less than 2 mm) generating little resistance to air movement given their overall cumulative large surface area and the diffusive nature of flow at these small airways' dimensions. Thus, the resistance of the smaller peripheral airways (less than 2 mm in internal diameter), where flow is laminar and surface area is large (average number of terminal bronchioles per lung approximately 25,000 in number), adds little to the total airflow resistance (McDonough 2011).

In the normal lung, these small peripheral airways (less than 2 mm in internal diameter) constitute only approximately 10–20 percent of total airway resistance. In normal, nondiseased subjects breathing spontaneously, Raw = 1.5–2.5 $cmH_2O/L/sec$. Similar values have been reported in patients free of lung disease on mechanical ventilation, equaling Raw = 2.2 $cmH_2O/L/sec$ at a flow rate of 0.6 L/sec, again noting the importance of including flow rate in the calculation of resistance to flow of any tubular structure, as already previously highlighted in section on upper-airway obstruction (UAO) (West 2005, Figure 7-14).

In critically ill patients without intrinsic lung disease and with non-lung-related respiratory failure, these same principles and numerical values apply. However, in virtually all airway-based diseases of the lung, such as asthma, chronic obstructive pulmonary disease (COPD), cystic fibrosis (CF), and bronchiolitis, a transition occurs whereby a progressively greater percentage of the Raw necessary for overcoming WOB moves downward into the small airways, which now, in these diseased states, become a significant resistive component of the WOB and can lead to excessive workloads such that acute respiratory failure (ARF) ensues (Hyatt 1961; Hogg 1968; Yanai 1992, Table 4 and Figure 5; McDonough 2011; Irvin 2011, Figure 1). Ineffective airway clearance, excessive mucus production, and airway mucoid impaction then contribute further to worsen the disease-induced abnormal lung physiology. Efforts at improving all of these components must then be undertaken to successfully improve the respiratory status of these now multifactor causes of increased Raw and resultant ARF.

Work of Breathing

Although compliance and resistance are often considered as "lumped" uniform parameters, in fact, marked regional differences exist in any clinical setting with significant inhomogeneity throughout the distribution of both healthy and diseased lungs (Marini 1989). Compliance, elastance, and resistance are primarily lung-derived physiological measurements and parameters with virtually no modulating factors resultant from patient overall non-lung-related health status such as multiorgan failure, muscular capacity, or overall endurance or strength—again noting that any episode of ARF is always a result of a combination and imbalance of these two clinical variables (i.e., WOB and respiratory muscle capacity). Thus, concepts of compliance expressed as $\Delta V/\Delta P$ (mL/cmH$_2$O) and Raw (cmH$_2$O/L/sec), being hard numbers, are somewhat easy to comprehend and are profiled on a regular basis in the care of ICU patients. However, the often nebulous entity of WOB is much more difficult to conceptualize and thus is discussed rarely on standard intensive-care unit (ICU) rounds in hard, exact terms, even though such factual data do indeed exist. Yet it is this entity (the WOB) that actually maintains and prolongs ventilator-dependent respiratory failure. Whether breathing spontaneously using active respiratory muscle effort or breathing passively, fully dependent upon mechanical ventilation, or *both*, work is required. The forces needed to be generated by the muscles of respiration during spontaneous breathing in healthy or diseased states or the pressures necessary to mechanically ventilate the lungs in cases of ARF follow these same principles and make up the combined forces that we cumulatively refer to as the WOB.

The WOB may be studied by measuring either (a) the total energy required by the respiratory muscles (O_2 cost of breathing) or (b) the mechanical work done by the respiratory muscles during spontaneous breathing or the mechanical energy provided by invasive ventilation (Leung 1997). The external mechanical work of breathing can be expressed in various numerical modalities: (a) external work per breath (Wbreath) expressed as Joules (J), (b) external work per liter of ventilation or volume (Wvol) expressed as (Wbreath/Vt) = J/L, or (c) external work per unit of time (Wtot) (Wbreath × RR) expressed as J/second, whereby 1 joule (J) = energy required to move 1 L of gas/air across/through a 10 cmH_2O pressure gradient (Cabello 2006; Cabello 2009).

Whatever the source of ventilatory power, whether patient, machine, or both, the mechanical work performed is computed as the pressure-volume product—that is, the integral of driving pressure and flow (Marini 1988; Marini 1989). When expressed mathematically, the WOB represents the integration of the area encompassed by the overall respiratory system P-V curve during the entire dynamic phase of inspiration that includes both compliance and resistance components (Otis 1964, Figure 5; Cabello 2009). The mechanical work expended during inflation of a passive structure over one cycle is defined as the integration of the product of the trans-structural distending pressure (P) and the rate of volume change ($\dot{V}$): $W = \int P\dot{V}\,dt$ (Otis 1964; Haas 1995). During mechanical ventilation, the work performed by the ventilator can be partitioned into these same components: (a) elastic WOB = $\int(Palv - Ppl)\,\dot{V}\,dt + \int(Ppl - Patm)\,\dot{V}\,dt$ plus (b) resistance WOB = $\int(Pao - Palv)\,\dot{V}\,dt$. Thus the total mechanical WOB = $\int(Pao - Patm)\,\dot{V}\,dt$ (Truwit and Marini 1988).

During inspiration, the driving pressure for ventilation can be generated in three ways: (a) entirely by the ventilator as the generation of positive airway pressure during passive inflation, (b) entirely by the patient's respiratory muscles as unassisted spontaneous ventilation, or (c) any combination of the two. During inspiration, respiratory WOB performed by either the respiratory muscles (Pmus) or the mechanical ventilator (Pvent) can be calculated in the same way by taking the integration or the area under the curve of the respiratory P-V relationship/curve (Roussos 1985; Roussos 1986, Figure 13; Truwit and Marini 1988, Figure 2; Banner 1994).

From both a descriptive and a visual understanding, the WOB is also often depicted in graphic display representing intrapleural or transpulmonary pressure versus volume expansion referenced as a percentage of tidal volume. Such a graphic representation is referred to as a Campbell diagram (Loring 2009; Banner 1994; Cabello 2009). A visual depiction of the effects of changes in lung mechanics, such as reduced compliance or increased Raw, can then be easily visualized by examining the requisite changes in transpulmonary pressure required to attain set values of lung expansion and tidal volume increase, again graphically represented as the areas under the P-V curve during dynamic phases of inspiration (Banner 1994, Figures 3, 4, 5, 6; Cabello 2009, Figure 1).

Under normal, healthy conditions and during spontaneous breathing, the normal energy expenditure for WOB approximates 0.25–0.75 J/L (Marini 1986; Banner 1994; Austin 2001) and can be mathematically partitioned into (a) 63.3 percent to overcome the elastic work of inspiration, (b) 28.5 percent to overcome the resistive component of inspiration, and (c) 8.2 percent to overcome the forces of tissue deformation during inspiration (Otis 1950).

Obviously, in the presence of disease, the absolute values for WOB will increase, and the percentage contributions will vary based upon the specific disease-related physiological abnormality. In a study of a mixed population of critically ill patients, various measurements of WOB demonstrated WOB_{lung} = 1.07 +/– 0.66 J/l; WOB_{cw} = 0.32 +/– 0.10 J/l; and WOB total = 1.39 +/– 0.68 J/l (Marini 1986). In a cohort of critically ill patients with a variety of causes of acute respiratory failure (including COPD, sepsis, and ARDS), the various components of total WOB can be partitioned into WOB patient and WOB ventilator, with values of WOB patient recorded as 0.52 +/– 0.34 J/L, 0.43 +/– 0.70 J/L, and 0.58 +/– 0.60 J/L and WOB vent recorded as 2.01 +/– 0.81J/L, 2.16 +/– 0.80 J/L, and 2.10 +/– 0.81J/L; the magnitude of patient-related WOB was highly dependent upon inspiratory flow rate (Haas 1995).

The measurement of absolute values for WOB is not simply a physiological phenomenon; it clearly has significant clinical impact. In general, a value for spontaneous WOB in excess of 1 J/L is believed to represent a value of energy expenditure that will often require the utilization of mechanical ventilatory assistance (Brochard 1989; Kallet 2011). In addition, one study demonstrated that serial measurements of WOB in a mixed population of critically ill patients during a spontaneous breathing trial (SBT) was highly predictive of extubation failure when the patient WOB measurement increased in magnitude greater than 0.12 J/L (Teixeira 2009; Kallet 2011, Figure 2).

Frequently, patient-assisted ventilation will continue throughout the entirety of the mechanical ventilator breath. In the context of limited respiratory reserve and muscle fatigue or weakness, the persistence of significantly elevated spontaneous patient WOB, even while receiving mechanical assistance, may be sufficient to prolong the need for invasive ventilation and significantly forestall successful weaning. In fact, multiple studies have demonstrated substantial levels of spontaneous patient-generated inspiratory WOB at virtually all levels and all modalities of ventilatory mechanical support in the absence of high-level sedation and/or paralysis (Sassoon 1994; Leung 1997; Aslanian 1998).

In a study of patients receiving synchronized intermittent mandatory ventilation (SIMV) as the mechanical mode of ventilation, the gradual reduction of levels of support during the weaning process demonstrated progressive increases in patient-specific WOB, often to levels above 1 J/L, with values that were not able to be sustained indefinitely (Marini 1988).

Alternatively, WOB can also be expressed in relation to the O_2 consumption of the respiratory muscles to achieve a set level of ventilation. The oxygen cost of breathing is an index of the total energy required by the respiratory muscles for ventilation. At rest, the oxygen cost of breathing is only 0.25–0.5 mLO_2/min per liter of ventilation or 1–2 percent of basal oxygen consumption (Collett 1988). In addition, during quiet, spontaneous breathing, the respiratory muscles receive only about 3 percent of the total cardiac output. During maximum respiratory efforts, during strenuous physical activity, the oxygen cost of breathing ($\dot{V}O_2$ resp) may reach 1,500 mL/min, and the predicted blood flow to the respiratory muscles may reach 10–15 L per minute (Collett 1988, Figure 4-24). In a group of critically ill patients with a variety of lung diseases requiring invasive mechanical ventilator support while undergoing a spontaneous breathing trial (SBT), $\dot{V}O_2$ resp measured 75 +/− 82 mLO$_2$/min (range 8–286) and $\dot{V}O_2$ resp/$\dot{V}O_2$ total measured 20% +/− 16 (range 6–55%) (Field 1982). Such excessive values of oxygen consumption utilization might not only limit the strength and endurance of the respiratory muscles as a factor toward weaning failure but also significantly reduce total body overall oxygen delivery (DO$_2$) to potentially threaten other vital organ tissue viability (Roussos 1985).

The pressure-time product (PTP) obtained during invasive mechanical ventilation is the analog of the tension-time index obtained in a spontaneously breathing individual and has been suggested as an indicator of oxygen consumption by the respiratory muscles in patients receiving mechanical ventilation. PTP is calculated similar to the P-V plots, except now using Pplat pressure versus time. In addition, the pressure-time index can also be calculated as the integral of esophageal pressure (Pes) tracing versus time during muscular inspiration and expressed as cmH$_2$O·sec. It can be expressed as either PTP per breath or PTP per minute (Imsand 1994; Jubran 1995; Cinnella 1996). Similar to estimates of WOB showing substantial activity spontaneously and excessive values in patients with prolonged ventilator-dependent respiratory failure (VDRF), measurements of the inspiratory PTP during reduced levels of mechanical assistance have also been shown to be predictive of ventilatory muscle capacity and endurance during weaning trials.

An arbitrarily selected upper bound or threshold value of inspiratory PTP per minute less than 125 cmH$_2$O·sec/min appears to represent a desirable level of inspiratory effort during pressure support ventilation (PSV), which is equivalent to a TTi = 0.08. Values for PTP in excess of 125 cmH$_2$O·sec/min portend the need for continued mechanical ventilatory assistance (Leung 1977, Figure 2; Jubran 1995, Figure 2; Cinnella 1996, Figure 4).

References

Amato, M.B.P., M.O. Meade, A.S. Slutsky, L. Brochard, E.L.V. Costa, D.A. Schoenfeld, T.E. Stewart, et. al. 2015. "Driving Pressure and Survival in the Acute Respiratory Distress Syndrome." *New England Journal of Medicine* 372: 747-755.

Aslanian, P., S. E. L. Atrous, D. Isabey, E. Valente, D. Corsi, A. Harf, F. Lemaire, and L. Brochard. 1998. "Effects of Flow Triggering on Breathing Effort during Partial Ventilator Support." *American Journal of Respiratory and Critical Care Medicine* 157: 135–143.

Austin, P. N., R. S. Campbell, J.A. Johannigman, and R. D. Branson. 2001. "Work of Breathing Characteristics of Seven Portable Ventilators." *Resuscitation* 49: 159–167.

Banner, M. J., M. J. Jaeger, and R. R. Kirby. 1994. "Components of the Work of Breathing and Implications for Monitoring Ventilator Dependent Patients." *Critical Care Medicine* 22 (3): 515–523.

Brochard, L., A. Harf, H. Lorino, and F. Lemaire. 1989. "Inspiratory Pressure Support Prevents Diaphragmatic Fatigue during Weaning from Mechanical Ventilation." *American Review of Respiratory Disease* 139: 513–521.

Cabello, B., and J. Mancebo. 2006. "Work of Breathing." *Intensive Care Medicine* 32: 1311–1314.

Cabello, B., and J. Mancebo. 2009. "Work of Breathing." In *Applied Physiology in Intensive Care Medicine*, edited by M. R. Pinsky et al. Dordrecht: Springer. 11–13.

Chatburn, R. L. 2006. "Classification of Mechanical Ventilators." In *Principles and Practice of Mechanical Ventilation*, edited by M. J. Tobin. New York: McGraw-Hill, Medical Publishing Division. 37–52.

Chiumello, D., E. Carlesso, P. Cadringher, P. Caironi, F. Valenza, F. Polli, F. Tallarini, P. Cozzi, M. Cressoni, A. Colombo, J. J. Marini, and L. Gattinoni. 2008. "Lung Stress and Strain during Mechanical Ventilation for Acute Respiratory Distress Syndrome." *American Journal of Respiratory and Critical Care Medicine* 178: 346–355.

Cinnella, G., G. Conti, F. Lofaso, H. Lorino, A. Harf, F. Lemaire, and L. Brochard. 1996. "Effects of Assisted Ventilation on the Work of Breathing: Volume Controlled versus Pressure Controlled Ventilation." *American Journal of Respiratory and Critical Care Medicine* 153: 1025–1033.

Collett, P. W., C. Roussos, and P. T. Macklem. 1988. "Respiratory Mechanics." In *Textbook of Respiratory Medicine*, edited by J. F. Murray and J. A. Nadel. Philadelphia: W. B. Saunders Company. 85–128.

Dhand, R., A. Jubran, and M. J. Tobin. 1995. "Bronchodilator Delivered by Metered-Dose Inhaler in Ventilator Supported Patients." *American Journal of Respiratory and Critical Care Medicine* 151: 1827–1833.

Fernandez-Perez, E. R., and R. D. Hubmayr. 2006. "Interpretation of Airway Pressure Waveforms." *Intensive Care Medicine* 32: 658–659.

Field, S., S. M. Kellu, and P. T. Macklem. 1982. "The Oxygen Cost of Breathing in Patients with Cardiorespiratory Disease." *American Review of Respiratory Disease* 126: 9–13.

Fishman, A. P. 1998. "Appendix C-4." In *Fishman's Pulmonary Diseases and Disorders*, edited by J. A. Elias et al. New York: McGraw-Hill, Health Professions Division. C-4.

Gattinoni, L., P. Caironi, M. Cressoni, D. Chiumello, V. M. Ranier, M. Quintel, S. Russo, N. Patroniti, R. Cornejo, and G. Bugedo. 2006.

"Lung Recruitment in Patients with the Acute Respiratory Distress Syndrome." *New England Journal of Medicine* 354 (17): 1775–1786.

Grimby, G., G. Hedenstierna, and B. Lofstrom. 1975. "Chest Wall Mechanics during Artificial Ventilation." *Journal of Applied Physiology* 38 (4): 576–580.

Grippi, M. A., L. F. Metzger, A. V. Sacks, A. P. Fishman, et al. 1998. "Pulmonary Function Testing." In *Fishman's Pulmonary Diseases and Disorders*, edited by J. A. Elias et al., 533–574. New York: McGraw-Hill, Health Professions Division.

Haas, C. F., R. D. Branson, L. M. Folk, R. S. Campbell, C. R. Wise, K. Davis, R. E. Dechert, and J. G. Weg. 1995. "Patient Determined Inspiratory Flow during Assisted Mechanical Ventilation." *Respiratory Care* 40 (7): 716–721.

Hess, D. R. 2014. "Respiratory Mechanics in Mechanically Ventilated Patients." *Respiratory Care* 59 (11): 1773–1794.

Hogg, J. C., P. T. Macklem, and W. M. Thurlbeck. 1968. "Site and Nature of Airway Obstruction in Chronic Obstructive Lung Disease." *New England Journal of Medicine* 278 (5): 1355–1360.

Hyatt, R. E., and R. E. Wilcox. 1961. "Extrathoracic Airway Resistance in Man." *Journal of Applied Physiology* 16 (2): 326–330.

Imsand, C., F. Feihl, C. Perret, and J. W. Fitting. 1994. "Regulation of Inspiratory Neuromuscular Output during Synchronized Intermittent Mechanical Ventilation." *Anesthesiology* 80 (1): 13–22.

Irvin, C. G. 2011. "Will the Small Airways Rise Again?" *American Journal of Respiratory and Critical Care Medicine* 184: 499–500.

Jubran, A., and M. J. Tobin. 1996. "Monitoring During Mechanical Ventilation." *Clinics in Chest Medicine* 17 (3): 453–473.

Jubran, A., W. B. Van de Graaff, M. J. Tobin. 1995. "Variability of Patient Ventilator Interaction with Pressure Support Ventilation in Patients with Chronic Obstructive Pulmonary Disease." *American Journal of Respiratory and Critical Care Medicine* 152: 129–136.

Kallet, R. H. 2011. "Patient-Ventilator Interaction during Acute Lung Injury, and the Role of Spontaneous Breathing: Part 1: Respiratory Muscle Function during Critical Illness." *Respiratory Care* 56 (2): 181–189.

Katz, J. A., S. E. Zinn, G. M. Ozanne, and H. B. Fairley. 1981. "Pulmonary, Chest Wall, and Lung-Thorax Elastances in Acute Respiratory Failure." *Chest* 80 (3): 304–311.

Leung, P., A. Jubran, and M. J. Tobin. 1997. "Comparison of Assisted Ventilator Modes on Triggering, Patient Effort, and Dyspnea." *American Journal of Respiratory and Critical Care Medicine* 55: 1940–1948.

Loring, S. H., M. Garcia-Jacques, and A. Malhotra. 2009. "Pulmonary Characteristics in COPD and Mechanism of Increased Work of Breathing." *Journal of Applied Physiology* 107 (1): 309–314.

Marini, J. J., P. S. Crooke, and J. D. Truwit. 1989. "Determinants and Limits of Pressure-Preset Ventilation: A Mathematical Model of Pressure Control." *Journal of Applied Physiology* 67 (3): 1081–1092.

Marini, J. J., R. M. Rodriguez, and V. Lamb. 1986. "The Inspiratory Workload of Patient-Initiated Mechanical Ventilation." *American Review of Respiratory Disease* 134: 902–909.

Marini, J. J., T. C. Smith, and V. J. Lamb. 1988. "External Work Output and Force Generation during Synchronized Intermittent Mechanical Ventilation." *American Review of Respiratory Disease* 138: 1169–1179.

McDonough, J. E., R. Yuan, M. Suzuki, N. Seyednejad, W. M. Elliott, P. G. Sanchez, A. C. Wright, et al. 2011. "Small Airway Obstruction and Emphysema in Chronic Obstructive Pulmonary Disease." *New England Journal of Medicine* 365: 1567–1575.

Neto, A.S., S. N. T. Hemmes, C.S.V. Barbas, M. Beiderlinden, A.F. Fernandez-Bustamante, E. Futier, O. Gajic, et. al. 2016. "Association Between Driving Pressure and Development of Postoperative Pulmonary Complications in Patients Undergoing Mechanical Ventilation for General Anesthesia: A Meta-analysis of Individual Patient Data." *Lancet Respiratory Medicine* 4: 272-280.

Otis, A. B. 1964. "The Work of Breathing." In *Handbook of Physiology: A Critical, Comprehensive Presentation of Physiological Knowledge and Concepts: Section 3, Volume 1.* American Physiological Society. Baltimore: Waverly Press, Inc. Distributed by the Williams & Wilkins Company. 463–476.

Otis, A. B., W. O. Fenn, and H. Rahn. 1950. "Mechanics of Breathing in Man." *Journal of Applied Physiology* 2: 592–607.

Rittayamai, N., C. M. Katsios, F. Beloncie, J. O. Friedrich, J. Mancebo, and L. Brochard. 2015. "Pressure-Controlled vs Volume-Controlled Ventilation in Acute Respiratory Failure: A Physiology-Based Narrative and Systematic Review." *Chest* 148(2): 340–355.

Roussos, C. 1985. "Energetics." In *Lung Biology in Health and Disease: The Thorax*, edited by C. Roussos and P. T. Macklem. New York: Marcel-Dekker, Inc. 437–492

Roussos, C., and E. J. J. M. Campbell. 1986. "Respiratory Muscle Energetics." In *Handbook of Physiology*. American Physiological Society. American Physiological Society. Baltimore: Waverly Press, Inc. Distributed by the Williams & Wilkins Company. 481–509.

Sassoon, C. S. H., N. Del Rosario, R. Fei, C. H. Rheeman, S. E. Gruer, and C. Kees Mahutte. 1994. "Influence of Pressure and Flow Triggered Synchronous Intermittent Mandatory Ventilation on Inspiratory Muscle Work." *Critical Care Medicine* 22 (12): 1933–1941.

Schlobohm, R. M., R. T. Falltrick, S. F. Quan, and J. A. Katz. 1981. "Lung Volumes, Mechanics, and Oxygenation during Spontaneous Positive Pressure Ventilation: The Advantage of CPAP over EPAP." *Anesthesiology* 55: 416–422.

Sharp, J. T., J. P. Henry, S. K. Sweany, W. R. Meadows, and R. J. Pietras. 1964. "The Total Work of Breathing in Normal and Obese Men." *Journal of Clinical Investigation* 43 (4): 728–739.

Sharp, J. T., and M. D. Hammond. 1991. "Pressure-Volume Relationships." In *The Lung Scientific Foundations*, edited by R. G. Crystal and J. B. West. New York: Raven Press. 839–854.

Singer, B. D., and T. C. Corbridge. 2009. "Basic Invasive Mechanical Ventilation." *Southern Medical Journal* 102 (12): 1238–1245.

Teixeira, C., P. J. Zimermann Teixeira, P. Pickersgill de Leon, and E. Silvestre Oliveira. 2009. "Work of Breathing during Successful Spontaneous Breathing Trial." *Journal of Critical Care* 24: 508–514.

Tobin, M. J. 1988. "Respiratory Monitoring in the Intensive Care Unit." *American Review of Respiratory Disease* 138: 1625–1642.

Tobin, M. J. 1990. "Respiratory Monitoring." *JAMA* 264 (2): 244–251.

Truwit, J. D., and J. J. Marini. 1988. "Evaluation of Thoracic Mechanics in the Ventilated Patient. Part II: Applied Mechanics." *Journal of Critical Care* 3 (3): 199–213.

Ward, M. E., C. Roussos, and P. T. Macklem. 1994. "Respiratory Mechanics." In *Textbook of Respiratory Medicine*, edited by J. F. Murray and J. A. Nadel. Philadelphia: W. B. Saunders Company. 90–138.

Warner, D. O. 2000. "So You Want to Be a Pulmonary Mechanic: A Clinical Guide." *Journal of Clinical Monitoring and Computing* 16: 417–423.

Weinberger, S. E., and J. M. Drazen. 1998. "Disturbances of Respiratory Function." In *Harrison's Principles of Internal Medicine*, edited by A. S. Fauci et al., 1410–1417. New York: McGraw-Hill, Health Professions Division.

West, J. B. 2005. "Mechanics of Breathing." In *Respiratory Physiology: The Essentials*. Philadelphia: Wolters Kluwer/Lippincott Williams & Wilkins. 93–120.

Yanai, M., K. Sekizawa, T. Ohrui, H. Sasaki, and T. Takishima. 1992. "Site of Airway Obstruction in Pulmonary Disease: Direct Measurement of Intrabronchial Pressure." *Journal of Applied Physiology* 72: 1016–1023.

CHAPTER 8

Pulmonary Circulation

• • •

ANATOMICALLY, THE PULMONARY CIRCULATION CAN be divided into the large conducting pulmonary arteries, the small intraparenchymal pulmonary arterioles, the alveolar capillaries (internal diameter of approximately 5–10 microns), and the venous system returning oxygenated blood to the left side of the heart. The resistance or stop-cock vessels of the pulmonary circulation constitute the small muscular pulmonary arterioles (50–500 microns in diameter). Physiological abnormalities of the pulmonary circulation can be manifest hemodynamically as pulmonary arterial hypertension (PAH) and resultant acute/chronic right heart failure and/ or abnormalities of gas exchange. Under normal, healthy circumstances, the largest component of resistance within the pulmonary circulation lies within the capillaries of the alveolar septum; however, from a disease perspective, it is the precapillary pulmonary arterioles (25–150 microns in diameter) that become the manifest site of pathology and abnormal pathophysiology resulting in PAH (Murray 1988).

The pulmonary circulation is a low-resistance, low-pressure, and low-impedance but high-capacitance, high-compliance, high-flow circulatory system receiving equal cardiac output as the systemic circulation but with a resting pulmonary arterial pressure (PAP) of only 25/10 mmHg (mean 15 mmHg). In addition, in the absence of pulmonary vascular disease, despite marked increases in flow as commonly occurs with disease, activity, and exercise, rarely does the PAP increase above a mean of 25 mmHg (Voelkel 1979, Figure 9). Part of this pressure-buffering effect is resultant from the fact that approximately 25 percent of the pulmonary circulation under healthy conditions is unperfused or underperfused and can be recruited in situations of increased stress, as manifested by increased flow (Glazier 1969). In addition, the low resistance of the pulmonary resistance arterioles allows for some degree of vasodilatation to accommodate portions of this increased flow without any significant concomitant increase in PAP.

Similar to other physiological processes, as the pulmonary vascular arterial density or surface area becomes reduced, this remarkable adaptability of the pulmonary circulation can still accommodate approximately 50 percent loss in pulmonary vascular surface area without any hemodynamic complications and any resultant elevation in either pulmonary vascular resistance (PVR) or PAP (Massion 1964, Figure 3; Petitpretz 1984, Figure 2). However, again, similar to other physiological processes, once the vascular bed becomes reduced below the remaining critical volume of approximately 40–50 percent of normal, exponential increases in pulmonary vascular resistance (PVR) and, consequently, PAP occur with even minor/trivial further reductions in arterial vascular volume or surface area. Obviously, in the presence of pulmonary vascular disease and existent reductions in pulmonary vascular surface area in association with fixed PVR resultant from anatomic structural changes (vasoconstriction), coupled with the inability to vasodilate or recruit additional vascular volumes or surface area, any situation of increased pulmonary blood flow and increased cardiac output (CO) will directly and linearly be transmitted with resultant marked increases in PAP, again noting the mathematical derivation of mean pulmonary arterial pressure (mPAP); that is, mPAP = (PVR × CO) + left atrial pressure (LAP).

Eventually, in association with pulmonary vascular disease (PVD) progression and resultant loss of all the pulmonary circulatory adaptive mechanisms, a point is reached when this pressure overload compensation by the right ventricle fails, and the right ventricle can no longer keep up with the pressure demands; and as CO drops, PAP drops in the same magnitude (remembering mPAP = [CO × PVR] + LAP), thus negating measurements of PAP alone as an indicator of either improvement or worsening of hemodynamic status in both acute and chronic medical conditions that cause pulmonary arterial hypertension. Thus, measurements of RV function, such as CO or right atrial pressure (RAP), are much more predictable indicators of prognosis and survival. RV function remains the most important determinant of morbidity and mortality for patients with any form of pulmonary hypertension (PH) (Bogaard 2012). In fact, for any pulmonary vascular disease causing either acute or chronic elevations in PVR, it is the right ventricular (RV) adaptive response to this increased pressure load, as assessed by cardiac output (CO), cardiac index (CI), right ventricle end-diastolic pressure (RVEDP), and right atrial pressure (RAP), that correlates best with outcome and mortality (Porhownik 2007, Figure 1; Simon 2010).

The corollary of these physiological principles is that any elevation, however minor, in PVR and subsequently PAP already represents significant and often late disease severity, and thus any degree of elevation in PVR above the normal calculated value of one to two units is clinically significant. In addition, in situations of acute pulmonary hypertension, the survivability of the patient is dependent upon the capacity of the RV to compensate and increase flow to maintain systemic perfusion despite the loss of significant volumes or profusion of pulmonary vascular surface area and consequent increase in PVR (Hoeper 2011). However, it is naïve and simplistic to think that PVR is the only factor contributing to any increased RV load. Additional variables only recently coming into consideration and evaluation include abnormalities in pulmonary arterial compliance, impedance, and stiffness (Thenappan 2016).

Pulmonary hypertension (PH) is defined as a resting mean pulmonary artery pressure (mPAP) greater than 25 mmHg; however, pulmonary *arterial* hypertension (PAH) is defined by three distinct additional hemodynamic criteria: (a) again mPAP > 25 mmHg + (b) pulmonary capillary wedge pressure (PCWP) or left atrial pressure (LAP) < 15–17 mmHg + (c) pulmonary vascular resistance (PVR) > 3 Wood units (whereby PVR = [mPAP − PCWP]/CO).

The recognition of the difference between terminology for pulmonary hypertension (PH) and pulmonary arterial hypertension (PAH) is extremely important from a number of perspectives: (a) the realization that pulmonary hypertension (PH) and pulmonary arterial hypertension (PAH) are not specific diseases per se but rather both are the hemodynamic consequences of defined pathological disease states and conditions, (b) the diagnosis of PAH identifies the site of pulmonary vascular disease as causing the abnormal pulmonary vascular hemodynamics to the precapillary small resistance arterioles of the lung (pulmonary arteries of caliber 25–150 micron), and (c) the fact that disease of these small-sized resistance vessels are the only clinical entities for which FDA-approved pulmonary vascular vasodirected therapies are approved and indicated (referred to as WHO Group 1) (McLaughlin 2009).

Few acute airway or parenchymal diseases affect the pulmonary circulation with sufficient profusion and vascular density to result in pulmonary arterial hypertension; the exception to this is the acute respiratory distress syndrome (ARDS). ARDS is a heterogeneous/inhomogeneous disease causing diffuse capillary injury from either exogenous or endogenous injurious agents. Yet the volume of lung and, by definition, mandatory capillary damage is extensive enough and is frequently associated with abnormalities of in situ vascular thrombosis that elevations in PVR do develop. However, given the massive volume of the alveolar capillary system, these elevations in PAP are rarely drastic and only infrequently result in cor pulmonale acutely.

In relation to diseases of the pulmonary circulation (especially WHO group 1)that cause pulmonary arterial hypertension (PAH), there are both important similarities and important differences essential to understanding mechanisms of disease. The most important similarity is the contribution of the pulmonary vascular surface area (PVSA) or pulmonary vascular arterial volume in determining PVR and the resultant pressure load or impedance placed upon the right ventricle. As already noted, the normal physiological characteristics of the pulmonary circulation and the pulmonary vascular bed render a large degree of reserve both during high-level exercise and also during disease before any overt increase in PAP or PVR is evident. In general, an approximate greater than 50 percent reduction in PVSA is required before any increase (even minor) in PVR and, consequently, increase in PAP will occur. This large reserve is the reason that only a trivial 10 mmHg increase in mPAP above the normal value of 15 mmHg to a value of mPAP = 25 mmHg is defined as PH. However, as the clinical impact of any increase in PVR is really determined by the impact of the increased impedance against the RV and the RV acute or adaptive response to any increase in PVR, important differences between various disease entities causing PAH include the time or rate of PAH development, the adaptability of the RV to any increase in strain, and the presence or absence of concomitant cardiopulmonary disease (McIntyre 1974).

As an example, for patients without concomitant comorbid cardiovascular disease who develop an acute pulmonary embolism (PE), cardiac index is usually increased or normal so as to maintain systemic tissue perfusion, unless angiographic obstruction exceeds 50 percent or mPAP approaches 40 mmHg (McIntyre 1974). Given the low resistance / high capacitance of the pulmonary circulation, acute venothromboembolic disease (VTE) must abruptly occlude a large and significant proportion of the pulmonary arterial circulation to result in PH and acute right-heart failure. Estimates suggest that this requires a volume of blood-clot occlusion of the pulmonary vascular bed of at least 40–50 percent of the pulmonary vasculature. In addition, given the acute nature of VTE, the RV has not had a sufficient time frame to adapt and undergo hypertrophy to accommodate this reduced pulmonary vascular volume / pulmonary vascular surface area and thus, in essence, fails at what would be perceived as relatively low absolute values of PAP, with acute pressures rarely exceeding systolic PAP of 50 mmHg. Despite massive embolic obstruction (> 50%), patients without prior cardiopulmonary disease are generally unable to generate mPAP > 40 mmHg, which appears to be the maximal pressure a healthy RV can generate acutely (McIntyre 1971; McIntyre 1974; Wood 2002). This contrasts with other chronic pulmonary hypertensive vascular diseases such as congenital heart disease (CHD), where RV compensation can generate PAP systolic and mean values near systemic levels. When RV afterload increases gradually, RV adaptation occurs, but progressive obliteration of the pulmonary vascular bed inevitably results in RV failure once RV-adaptive mechanisms have been exhausted (Hoeper 2011). In fact, in relation to diseases resulting in PAH causing either acute or chronic elevations in PVR, the RV adaptive response to this increased pressure load (as assessed by CO, CI, RVEDP, and RAP) correlates best with outcomes and mortality.

These important differences are most evident in comparison of distinct and separate disease entities that both affect the pulmonary circulation and compromise the density of the PVSA—namely, (a) as previously noted, the relatively acute onset disease VTE and (b) the relatively slower-onset idiopathic-primary pulmonary arterial hypertension (IPAH) or PAH associated with congenital heart disease (CHD). In the presence of an acute massive increase in PVR, such as a consequence of acute major / large-volume clot-burden VTE, and given the absence of time or mechanisms for RV adaption, large reductions in PVSA (often greater than 40%) can result in clinical shock, RV failure, and often death, but yet mPAP rarely exceeds 40-50 mmHg. This contrasts with the relatively longer duration and slower-onset disease process IPAH or CHD, wherein the gradual reductions in PVSA allow time for RV hypertrophy and adaptation. In these cases, marked increases in PAP may be observed, often close to systemic values with reasonably preserved patient functionality and the absence of shock.

Although life-threatening PE has traditionally been equated with anatomic vascular obstruction (>50%), it seems reasonable to assume that the clinical outcome is, in reality, a combination relating to the interaction of the acute event and underlying cardiopulmonary function, whose factors form the basis for the current classification of hemodynamic severity of acute PE as massive or submassive, determined by clinical factors or indices such as blood pressure, shock, or hypotension rather than based upon any absolute measurement of PAP (McIntyre 1974). Thus, in relation to

VTE, the hemodynamic status is a much more reliable predictor of outcome than the degree of angiographic obstruction (Wood 2002).

Nevertheless, invasive hemodynamic studies of patients diagnosed with PE have shown a clear linear relationship between percent of angiographic vascular obstruction and mPAP and mean right atrial (mRA) pressure (McIntyre 1971). In one series of patients with acute PE and the absence of prior cardiopulmonary disease, percentage of angiographic occlusion demonstrated a mean value of 37 percent +/- 16 (range 13-68%) and mPAP = 26 +/- 9 mmHg (range 10-38) but reasonably preserved CI and mRAP (3.1 +/- 1.1 L/min and 7.5 +/- 4 mmHg, respectively) (McIntyre 1971). Similar to other pulmonary vascular diseases, and consistent with the understanding of the hemodynamic principles of the pulmonary circulation, another study demonstrated that the relationship between total pulmonary vascular resistance and the level of pulmonary vascular obstruction was nonlinear but showed a hyperbolic tendency with dramatic increases in resistances when vascular obstruction exceeded 60 percent (Petitpretz 1984, Figure 2).

REFERENCES

Bogaard, H. J., R. Natarajan, S. C. Henderson, C. S. Long, D. Kraskauskas, L. Smithson, R. Ockaili, J. M. McCord, and N. F. Voelkel. 2012. "Chronic Pulmonary Artery Pressure Elevation Is Insufficient to Explain Right Heart Failure." *Circulation* 120: 1951–1960.

Glazier, J. B., J. M. B. Hughes, J. E. Maloney, and J. B. West. 1969. "Measurements of Capillary Dimensions and Blood Volume in Rapidly Frozen Lungs." *Journal of Applied Physiology* 26 (1): 65–76.

Hoeper, M. M., and J. Granton. 2011. "Intensive Care Unit Management of Patients with Severe Pulmonary Hypertension and Right Heart Failure." *American Journal of Respiratory and Critical Care Medicine* 184: 1114–1124.

Massion, W. H., and J. A. Schilling. 1964. "Physiological Effects of Lung Resection in Adult and Puppy Dogs." *Journal of Thoracic and Cardiovascular Surgery* 48: 239–250.

McIntyre, K. M., and A. A. Sasahara. 1971. "The Hemodynamic Response to Pulmonary Embolism in Patients without Prior Cardiopulmonary Disease." *American Journal of Cardiology* 28: 288–294.

McIntyre, K. M., and A. A. Sasahara. 1974. "Determinants of Right Ventricular Function and Hemodynamics after Pulmonary Embolism." *Chest* 65 (5): 534–543.

McLaughlin, V. V., S. L. Archer, D. B. Badesch, R. J. Barst, H. W. Farber, J. R. Linder, M. A. Mathier, M. D. McGoon, M. H. Park, R. S. Rosenson, L. J. Rubin, V. F. Tapson, and J. Varga. 2009. "ACCF/AHA 2009 Expert Consensus Document on Pulmonary Hypertension." *Journal of the American College of Cardiology* 53: 1573–1619.

Murray, J. F. 2000. "Disorders of the Pulmonary Circulation." In *Textbook of Respiratory Medicine*, edited by J. F. Murray and J. A. Nadel. Philadelphia: Saunders Company. 1485–1502.

Petitpretz, P., G. Simmoneau, J. Cerrina, D. Musset, M. Dreyfus, M. Vandenbroek, and P. Duroux. 1984. "Effects of a Single Bolus of Urokinase in Patients with Life Threatening Pulmonary Emboli: A Descriptive Trial." *Circulation* 70 (5): 861–866.

Porhownik, N. R., and Z. Bshouty, Z. 2007. "Pulmonary Arterial Hypertension: A Serious Problem." *Perspectives in Cardiology* 23(4): 33–40.

Simon, M. A. 2010. "Right Ventricular Adaptation to Pressure Overload." *Current Opinions in Critical Care* 16: 237–243.

Thenappan, T., Prins, K. W., Pritzker, M. R., Scandurra, J., Volmers, K., Weir, and K. E. 2016. "The Critical Role of Pulmonary Arterial Compliance in Pulmonary Hypertension." *Annals of the American Thoracic Society.* 13: 276-284.

Voelkel, N., and J. T. Reeves. 1979. "Primary Pulmonary Hypertension." In *Pulmonary Vascular Diseases*, edited by K. M. Moser. New York: Marcel Dekker, Inc. 573–628

Wood, K. 2002. "Major Pulmonary Embolism: A Pathophysiological Approach to the Golden Hour of Hemodynamically Significant Pulmonary Embolism." *Chest* 121 (3): 877–905.

CHAPTER 9

Control of Ventilation and Central Respiratory Drive

• • •

THE CENTRAL NERVOUS SYSTEM (CNS) respiratory controllers are divided into the automatic, involuntary, chemically driven brainstem respiratory neuron group and the voluntary, or volitional, cerebral cortex respiratory-activating neuron group. Within the medulla, there are two dense bilaterally organized aggregates of respiratory neurons that exhibit phasic discharges locked to either the inspiration (I) or expiration (E) phase of the respiratory cycle. In the dorsal medial medulla, just ventrolateral to the solitary tract, is one of these aggregates of neurons termed the dorsal respiratory group (DRG). In the ventrolateral medulla is a much longer, longitudinally oriented column of cells associated with three separate nuclear groups. This second aggregate group of respiratory neurons is known as the ventral respiratory group (VRG) (Berger 1988, Figure 7-5; Cherniak 1991; Kazemi 1991; von Euler 1991).

Most neural activity recorded within animals from the area of the DRG is inspiratory, and only a small portion of expiratory activity is located in this site (Berger 1988). The VRG contains both I and E neurons, which are arranged along a longitudinal column that extends throughout the medulla. It should come as no surprise that the response of the central chemosensitive neurons to CO_2/H^+ involves multiple signaling pathways, but the most common and potent stimulus to ventilation is hypercapnic acidosis (Putnam 2004). The bulk of respiratory response to CO_2 arises from these chemoreceptors within the brain stem. Studies have shown that CO_2 is the dominant stimulus for central chemosensitive respiratory neurons, and their firing response is at least in part mediated by an increase in respiratory neuronal intracellular free protons—that is, decrease in intracellular pH (pHi) (Wiemann, 2005). In experimental animal studies, the firing rate of these neurons in response to acid challenge was best correlated with the magnitude and rate of fall in intracellular pH (pHi) (Wiemann 1998; Filosa 2002).

The only signal that could serve as an adequate stimulus is the change in pHi in response to increase minute ventilation secondary to hypercapnic acidosis (Putnam, 2004). With an increase in $PaCO_2$, there is an immediate and marked rise in ventilation. This is not the case for hypoxia. However, varying degrees of hypoxemia can clearly alter the slope and intensity of the ventilatory response to hypercapnic acidosis resulting from reflex stimulation of peripheral chemoreceptors (i.e., the carotid and aortic bodies). For any given level of hypoxemia, central ventilatory response to alveolar partial pressure of CO_2 ($PACO_2$) is augmented, and the more severe the degree of hypoxemia, the greater the magnitude of increased ventilatory response.

The total respiratory system $PaCO_2$ set point under normal resting conditions is then determined by the intersection of the CO_2 metabolic hyperbola (defined by the relationship of the chemical characteristics of CO_2 and the magnitude of V̇A) and the respiratory control system response to increases in $PACO_2$. This relationship is graphically displayed in the accompanying references (Berger 1988, Figure 7-1; Caruana-Montaldo, 2000).

The effector system for effective ventilation consists of those pathways and muscles involved in the actual performance of inspiratory (predominately the diaphragm and external intercostals) and expiratory muscle (predominately the internal intercostals and abdominals) activity. Both cortical- (voluntary) and medullary- (involuntary) stimulated respiratory central-drive signals and pathways descend into the spinal cord. The spinal pathways connect the central respiratory centers in the brain and spinal cord to the respiratory muscles and are divided into ascending and descending pathways. Two main separate and distinct descending pathways control the lower motor neurons that innervate the respiratory muscles—that is, the corticospinal pyramidal tract and the bulbospinal or reticulospinal tract. The corticospinal-pyramidal tract neurons originating from the motor cortex are responsible for voluntary control of breathing and are widely dispersed throughout the cortex but more concentrated when passing through the internal capsule. The reticulospinal tract originates from the CNS medullary center neurons in the brainstem. The phrenic motor nucleus consists of a long, narrow column of cells located in the most ventral aspect of the ventral horn and extends through several segments of the cervical spinal cord (Laghi 2003, Figure 12).

Clinically it is not possible to actually measure or quantify neuronal discharge or frequency originating from these CNS located respiratory neurons. However, P0.1 is the airway occlusion pressure (measured in cmH_2O) that is generated at the distal end of an endotracheal tube 0.1 seconds (100msec) after initiation of spontaneous breath and represents a noninvasive reproducible technique to indirectly assess the central respiratory drive (Montgomery 1987; Sassoon 1993). P0.1 appears to be an index of the output of the central respiratory system, which depends only on neuronal discharge and the effectiveness of contraction of the respiratory muscles (Whitelaw 1975). In healthy volunteers, P0.1 (cmH_2O) rises linearly in relation to $PaCO_2$ using rebreathing techniques (Whitelaw 1975).

Thus, the measurements of P0.1 have been used clinically as a surrogate of central respiratory drive in efforts to assess this parameter in critically ill patients, most commonly patients with severe COPD. In contrast to healthy control patients or subjects, patients with either clinically stable COPD (Celli 1997; Marin 1999) or patients with COPD requiring mechanical ventilation resulting from acute respiratory failure (Pourriat 1986; Pourriat 1992; Montgomery 1987), marked elevations in P0.1 have been recorded (Table 9.1). This data indicated that in the absence of sedation, primary neuromuscular diseases, and/or severe metabolic alkalosis, a reduction in CNS drive is not a factor limiting weaning or precipitating respiratory failure; rather, the increased central drive is in response to both acute and chronic increases in respiratory load as measured by excessive work of breathing (WOB). In addition, a complementary study demonstrated that the discharge frequencies of the diaphragmatic motor units recorded in patients admitted with acute exacerbations of COPD (AECOPD) averaged 18 Hz, which is unequivocal evidence that in relation to patients admitted with AECOPD, the neural drive to the diaphragm is markedly increased (De Troyer 1997; Jolley 2009).

Table 9.1 Values of P 0.1 (cmH_2O) in Healthy Subjects and Various Patient Populations

Healthy	Stable COPD	COPD weaning from mechanical ventilation	Mixed population critically ill-ventilated
1.4 +/− 0.4	3.4+/−1.8	8.86+/−3.09	3.7 +/− 0.7 (2.0–7.7)
1.32 +/− 0.45	2.35 +/− 1.24	6.93 +/− 2.82	5.7 +/− 1.4 (2.3–13.6)
(0.84–2.3)	(0.5–5.5)		

Although a rare disorder with an estimated worldwide incidence of approximately one thousand individuals, central congenital hypoventilation syndrome (CCHS) represents an illuminating example of the interplay and interaction of multiple neurological effector systems in CNS respiratory control, drive, and adaptation to multiple internal stimuli and exogenous agents. Although initially described as a pediatric-aged disease, often with catastrophic symptoms manifest within the first twenty-four hours of birth, CCHS is now being recognized, diagnosed, and managed in adulthood with increasing numbers of case reports and case series describing this unique characteristic cohort of patients with late-onset presentation.

CCHS is a disorder of respiratory control with related autonomic nervous system (ANS) dysregulation/dysfunction (Antic 2006). Children with CCHS have a complex phenotype reflective of the overall imbalance of the autonomic nervous system, thus stressing that CCHS is not simply a disease of abnormal respiratory control; other ANS abnormalities include decreased heart-rate variability, diminished pupillary light reflex response, poor temperature regulation with profuse sweating, esophageal and intestinal dysmotility, and an association with Hirschsprung disease and/or tumors of neural crest origin (Weese-Mayer 2004; Antic 2006).

The disease-defining gene for CCHS results from mutations in the PHOX2B gene located on chromosome 4p12 that codes for a highly conserved transcription factor known to play a key role in the development of the ANS (Antic 2006). PHOX2B remains highly expressed in neurons of the hindbrain involved in the chemical drive and reflex regulation of the respiratory rhythm generator in animals, and a similar role is extrapolated to humans also (Weese-Mayer 2010). As a tissue-specific transcription factor, PHOX2B is responsible for the expression regulation of a series of target genes involved in embryogenesis and development of the ANS (Weese-Mayer 2010). However, it is changes in the length of the twenty-five-repeat polyalanine expansion sequence in the PHOX2B gene that create disease manifestations. The vast majority of individuals with CCHS are heterozygous for this polylalanine repeat-expansion mutation involving the second polyalanine repeat sequence in exon 3 of PHOX2B. These expansions are in frame and range from fifteen to thirty-nine nucleotide insertions, resulting in the expansion of the normal twenty-repeat polylalanine tract to twenty-five to thirty-three repeats. Most expansion mutations occur de novo, but a small number of families segregating with diagnosis of CCHS demonstrate an autosomal dominant inheritance pattern (Berry-Kravis 2006). The length of the polyalanine expansion sequence and expansion size correlates with disease severity with an expansion size of twenty-five repeats appearing to be minimal mutation abnormality associated with phenotypic disease presentation (Antic 2006; Berry-Kravis 2006).

Alveolar hypoventilation is the hall mark symptom of CCHS and represents its most debilitating and potentially fatal phenotypic feature (Weese-Mayer 2010). Most severely affected children hypoventilate during both wakefulness and sleep, and in such severely affected individuals, tracheostomy and initiation of full-time, continuous mechanical ventilation is a required therapy. Adult-onset or late-onset CCHS patients usually have adequate ventilation during wakefulness but still require invasive mechanical ventilation during sleep. Patients diagnosed in adulthood frequently report clues during the childhood years that suggest the diagnosis of CCHS, again reflecting the major impact of this disease upon respiratory control, such as voluntary breath holding to point of developing significant hypercapnia or reports of being able to hold their breath and swim underwater for prolonged periods.

REFERENCES

Antic, N. A., B. A. Malow, N. Lange, R. D. McEvoy, A. L. Olson, P. Turkington, W. Windisch, M. Samuels, C. A. Stevens, E. M. Berry-Kravis, and D. E. Weese-Mayer. 2006. "PHOX2B Mutation-Confirmed Congenital Central Hypoventilation Syndrome: Presentation in Adulthood." *American Journal of Respiratory and Critical Care Medicine* 174 (8): 923–927.

Berger, A. J. 1998. "Control of Breathing." In *Textbook of Respiratory Medicine*, edited by J. F. Murray and J. A. Nadel. Philadelphia: W. B. Saunders Company. 149–168.

Berry-Kravis, E. M., L. Zhou, C. M. Rand, D. E. Weese-Mayer. 2006. "Congenital Central Hypoventilation Syndrome: PHOX2B Mutations and Phenotype." *American Journal of Respiratory and Critical Care Medicine* 174 (10): 1139–1144.

Caruana-Montaldo, B. and C. W. Zwillich. 2000. "The Control of Breathing in Clinical Practice." *Chest* 117: 205–225.

Celli, B. R., M. Montes de Oca, R. Mendez, J. Stetz. 1997. "Lung Reduction Surgery in Severe COPD Decreases Central Drive and Ventilator Response to CO_2." *Chest* 112: 902–906.

Cherniack, N. S. 1991. "Central Chemoreceptors." In *The Lung: Scientific Foundations*, edited by R. G. Crystal. New York: Raven Press. 1349–1357.

De Troyer, A., J. B. Leeper, D. K. McKenzie, S. C. Gandevia, et al. 1997. "Neural Drive to the Diaphragm In Patients with Severe COPD." *American Journal of Respiratory and Critical Care Medicine* 155: 1335–1340.

Filosa, J. A., J. B. Dean, R. W. Putnam. 2002. "Role of Intracellular and Extracellular pH in the Chemo-Sensitive Response of Rat Locus Coeruleus Neurons." *Journal of Physiology* 541: 493–509.

Jolley, C. J., Y-M. Luo, J. Steier, C. Reilly, J. Seymour, A. Lunt, K. Ward. G. F. Rafferty, M. I. Polkey, and J. Moxham. 2009. "Neural Respiratory Drive in Healthy Subjects and in COPD." *European Respiratory Journal* 33: 289–297.

Kazemi, H. 1991. "Cerebrospinal Fluid and the Control of Ventilation." In *The Lung: Scientific Foundations*, edited by R. G. Crystal. New York: Raven Press. 1359–1367.

Laghi, F., and M. J. Tobin. 2003. "Disorders of the Respiratory Muscles." *American Journal of Respiratory and Critical Care Medicine* 168: 10–48.

Marin, J. M., M. M. de Oca, J. Rassulo, B. R. Celli. "Ventilatory Drive at Rest and Perception of Exertional Dyspnea in Severe COPD." *Chest* 115: 1293–1300.

Montgomery, A. B., R. H. O. Holle, S. R. Neagley, D. J. Pierson, and R. B. Schoene. 1987. "Prediction of Successful Ventilator Weaning Using Airway Occlusion Pressure and Hypercapnic Challenge." *Chest* 91 (4): 496–499.

Pourriat, J. L., Ch. Lamberto, P. H. Hoang, J. L. Fournier, and B. Vasseur. 1986. "Diaphragmatic Fatigue and Breathing Pattern during Weaning from Mechanical Ventilation in COPD Patients." *Chest* 90 (5): 703–707.

Pourriat, J. L., M. Baud, C. Lamberto, J. P. Fosse, and M. Cupa. 1992. "Effects of Doxapram on Hypercapnic Response during Weaning from Mechanical Ventilation in COPD Patients." *Chest* 101 (6): 1639–1643.

Putnam, R. W., J. A. Filosa, N. A. Ritucci. 2004. "Cellular Mechanisms Involved in CO_2 and Acid Signaling in Chemosensitive Neurons." *American Journal of Physiology: Cell Physiology* 287: C1493–C1526.

Sassoon, C. S. H., and C. K. Mahutte. 1993. "Airway Occlusion Pressure and Breathing Pattern as Predictors of Weaning Outcome." *American Review of Respiratory Disease* 148: 860–866.

Von Euler, C. 1991. "Neural Organization and Rhythm Generation." In *The Lung: Scientific Foundations*, edited by R. G. Crystal. New York: Raven Press. 1307–1318.

Weese-Mayer, D. E., and E. M. Berry-Kravis. 2004. "Genetics of Congenital Central Hypoventilation Syndrome: Lessons from Seemingly Orphan Disease." *American Journal of Respiratory Critical Care Medicine* 170 (1): 16–21.

Weese-Mayer, D. E., E. M. Berry-Kravis, I. Ceccherini, T. G. Keens, D. A. Loghmanee, and H. Trang. 2010. "An Official ATS Clinical Policy Statement: Congenital Central Hypoventilation Syndrome; Genetic Basis, Diagnosis, and Management." *American Journal of Respiratory Critical Care Medicine* 181 (6): 626–644.

Whitelaw, W. A., J. P. Derenne, and J. Milic-Emili. 1975. "Occlusion Pressure as a Measure of Respiratory Center Output in Conscious Man." *Respiratory Physiology* 23: 181–199.

Wiemann, M., R. E. Baker, U. Bonnet, D. Bingmann. 1998. "CO_2-Sensitive Medullary Neurons: Activation by Intracellular Acidification." *NeuroReport* 9: 167–170.

Wiemann, M., S. Frede, D. Bingmann, P. Kiwull, and H. Kiwull-Schone. 2005. "Sodium/Proton Exchangers in the Medulla Oblongata and Set Point of Breathing Control. *American Journal of Respiratory Critical Care Medicine* 172: 244–249.

CHAPTER 10

Respiratory Muscles

• • •

VENTILATION, WHICH INCLUDES LUNG INFLATION and chest-wall expansion, requires muscular effort/work in spontaneously breathing individuals and mechanical ventilator work for intubated patients requiring invasive mechanical support. The movement of air into the lung during inspiration requires the creation of pressure gradients to effect flow and then volume expansion. Air moves in and out of the lungs whenever the sum of pressures developed by passive recoil of the respiratory system and by the respiratory muscles (or mechanical ventilation) is other than zero. During spontaneous breathing, the actions of the inspiratory muscles cause an increase in the outward recoil of the chest wall; as a result, pleural pressure becomes reduced relative to atmospheric pressure (i.e., subatmospheric). This pressure change is transmitted to the interior of the lungs so alveolar pressure also becomes subatmospheric, thus the term "negative pressure ventilation." Of all the inspiratory muscles, the most significant in healthy humans is the diaphragm, which, during quiet respiration, accounts for 70–80 percent of lung volume change. The extradiaphragmatic inspiratory muscles include the scalene, parasternal intercostals, and the sternocleidomastoids.

Diaphragm muscle fibers radiate from a central tendinous structure (the central tendon) that inserts peripherally onto (a) the ventrolateral aspect of the first three lumbar vertebrae and the aponeurotic acruate ligament and (b) the costal portion onto the xiphoid process of the sternum and upper margins of the lower six ribs. The diaphragm is innervated by the cervical nerve roots at C3 through C5 and abuts the lower ribcage in a region referred to as the zone of apposition. When tension increases within the diaphragmatic muscle fibers, a caudally oriented force is then applied on the central tendon such that the dome of the diaphragm descends, the abdominal contents are displaced caudally, and abdominal pressure increases in the zone of apposition, and the lower ribcage expands. During spontaneous ventilation, when the diaphragm contracts, its insertions are pulled toward its origin, flattening the diaphragm dome, increasing the vertical dimensions of the thoracic cavity, increasing the volume of the thorax along its craniocaudal axis (causing intrathoracic pressure to fall), and reducing alveolar pressure (Palv) below barometric pressure (Pb) or mouth pressure (Pmouth).

The respiratory muscles—and most importantly the diaphragm, which is the primary muscle of inspiration—are skeletal muscles similar to those of the extremities. Similar to the muscles of the extremities, the respiratory muscles, again focusing on the diaphragm, must overcome a load expressed as the work of breathing (WOB), which, if excessive, can lead to fatigue and overt respiratory failure. However, the diaphragm is unique in that, as opposed to other skeletal muscles whose primary function is to provide movement and overcome inertia, the diaphragm's primary function is respiration, whose primary factor is to overcome resistive and elastic loads. The mechanical action of any skeletal muscle is determined by its unique (a) anatomy, (b) physiology, and (c) load. From basic physiology, the force generated by muscle contraction is related to the number of fibers stimulated, the frequency of stimulation, the muscle length at the time of stimulation, and the degree of freedom for movement (Polkey 2001).

The diaphragm manifests both voluntary and involuntary neural inputs and must contract rhythmically and continuously, as the respiratory muscles are the only skeletal muscles upon which life depends. To accomplish this role, the diaphragm consists of a unique mixture of muscle fibers adapted to be responsive to the above noted factors consisting of (a) 55 +/− 5 percent of type I fibers (high endurance), (b) 21+/− 6 percent of type IIa fibers (fast twitch / fatigue resistant), and (c) 23+/− 3 percent type IIb fibers (fast twitch / fatigable) (Decramer 1988). It is the specific muscle fiber composition plus the relatively large capillary density that allows the diaphragm to function continuously and, in most situations, efficiently to sustain life and allow requisite levels of ventilation to achieve and sustain exertion and activity. Being skeletal in nature, the diaphragm and other respiratory muscles also are subject to the same physiological characteristics of skeletal muscles in general, most specifically the fact that maximal tension is generated by an ideal or optimal length-tension relationship. Its aberration, in terms of reducing diaphragm strength, is most evident in cases of emphysema and lung air trapping plus chest-wall hyperinflation, which shortens the length-tension relationship of the diaphragm and reduces force-generating capacity, thus limiting extent of respiratory muscle induced endurance ventilation. Under healthy conditions, the diaphragm is well adapted to perform the continuous rhythmic contractions vital to survival. However, like all skeletal muscles, limits and restrictions to this contractility exist both as a result of disease and also as a result of systems overload, either of which can precipitate respiratory failure or death.

The action of the diaphragm is to lower pressure within the thorax and to raise pressure within the abdomen. The ability of the diaphragm to lower intrathoracic pressure is estimated by measurement of esophageal pressure (Pes). The most widely reported measure of diaphragm strength is the transdiaphragmatic pressure (Pdi), calculated as the difference between gastric pressure (Pga) and Pes; that is, Pdi = Pga − Pes. Pdimax is obtained during a maximal inspiratory effort. In general, healthy adult men can generate a Pdimax approximately 115 +/− 27 cmH$_2$O, with values measured in women approximately 25 percent lower and with values for both genders decreasing with age.

Under healthy, restful-breathing conditions, the ratio of Pdi/Pdimax is approximately 20 percent; Pdi/Pdimax values greater than 40 percent cannot be tolerated indefinitely without the onset of muscular fatigue (duration less than forty-five minutes) and will eventually result in respiratory failure if not relieved of this ventilatory load (Pourriat 1986; Mador 1991). Thus an increase in inspiratory load (by increasing the required Pdi to maintain ventilation) and/or decrease in inspiratory muscle strength (by decreasing Pdi or Pdimax) will then predispose to the development of fatigue (Roussos 1977, Figure 3 and Figure 4; Kelsen 1988).

Skeletal muscle **fatigue** must be differentiated from skeletal muscle weakness. Fatigue is defined as the loss in muscle capacity to develop force or to shorten resulting from muscle fiber activity under a load that is *reversible with rest*. Muscle fatigue can be defined as the loss of contractile function—force, velocity, power, or work—caused by prolonged exercise and/or excessive loads and reversible by rest (Aubier et al. 1990). Contractile fatigue is a reversible impairment in the contractile response to neural impulses in an overloaded muscle (Mador 1991). Consequences of fatigue include (a) depressed force generation and (b) reduced velocity of shortening. Contractile fatigue occurs when a sufficiently large respiratory load is supplied over a sufficiently long period, which, in relation to the diaphragm, can be depicted as Pdi/Pdimax (i.e., load) and Ti/Ttot (which is termed the diaphragmatic duty time that represents the amount of time that the diaphragm is maintained in active contraction).

Skeletal muscle **weakness** is defined as the impairment in the capacity of a *fully rested* muscle to generate force (Kelsen 1988; Mador 1991). Although both factors (weakness and fatigue) have important relevance for patients with a variety of causes of acute respiratory failure (ARF), this differentiation is important in relation to therapies and clinical outcomes. Muscle fatigue tends to result from stress, overuse, and metabolic factors, whereas muscle weakness tends to result from pathological neuromuscular disease states such as Guillain-Barre syndrome (GBS), myasthenia gravis (MG), or amyotrophic lateral sclerosis (ALS).

In addition, the duty time (i.e., Ti/Ttot) of ventilation (time spent in muscular inspiratory effort) also can result in respiratory muscle fatigue. This is because increases in Ti/Ttot will automatically increase the duration of diaphragm contraction relative to the period that the diaphragm as a muscle exists in its relaxed state such that resultant marked increases in Ti/Ttot will hasten the onset of diaphragm fatigue at any given ratio of

Pdi/Pdimax. For any given Pdi/Pdimax, the shorter the time that the diaphragm remains in active contraction (Ti) in relation to the total breathing cycle (Ttot)—that is, the duty time—then the smaller Ti/Ttot will result in the longer endurance time (Tlim) (Roussos 1977; Bellemare 1982; Kelsen 1988).

Not surprisingly, then, the ability of the respiratory muscle to sustain an increase in inspiratory load without onset of fatigue has been shown to be reliably predicted based upon the product of these two physiological variable ratios (i.e., the Ti divided by Ttot and the mean Pdi divided by Pdimax). The product of these two ratios is termed the tension-time index (i.e., TTi = Ti/Ttot × Pdi/Pdimax). A TTi of less than 0.15 can be maintained indefinitely, whereas a TTi greater than 0.18 leads to task failure within a finite period. Thus, the inspiratory muscle fatigue thresholds occur at TTi between 0.15 and 0.18 (Mador 1991). Healthy subjects at rest generally have a TTi of 0.02, which represents an eight- to ninefold reserve before task failure. Stable COPD patients have TTi approximately 0.05 (range 0.01–0.12) during restful breathing, but to accomplish this, COPD patients require a mean twofold higher discharge frequency from the phrenic nerve motor neurons and subsequent respiratory muscle activation (Bellemare 1982, Figure 4).

In the critical-care setting, innumerable factors can precipitate diaphragm muscle fatigue, some factors dependent upon lung mechanics and others independent. Aging, malnutrition, and electrolyte abnormalities are examples of nonlung factors that can precipitate fatigue. Increased WOB generated by any factor that increases ventilatory impedance or resistance or that increase ventilatory drive with concomitant effects upon the diaphragm tension-time index can precipitate fatigue (Cinnella 1996).

Endurance reflects the ability of a muscle to sustain mechanical output during loaded contraction and the muscle capacity to resist fatigue (ATS/ERS 1999). The time to task failure (i.e., endurance time) is also closely related to the requisite oxygen cost of breathing. For any given ventilatory load, the greater the oxygen cost of breathing, the shorter the endurance time (Mador 1991).

Acknowledging the aforementioned mechanical stresses upon diaphragm function, and again recognizing the similarity to any skeletal muscle, the force-generating capacity of the diaphragm is also dependent upon a sufficient supply of nutrients and oxygen to meet metabolic demands (Altose 1998). At resting ventilation, the total blood flow to the muscles of respiration is only 1.5 percent of the cardiac output, but at increased levels of added resistance, this fraction rises exponentially to 10.6 percent. Normal range for $V\dot{}O_2$ respiratory muscles in healthy, non-diseased individuals measured 0.25–2.5 mL O_2/minute/L (1–4% of total body $V\dot{}O_2$) (Collett 1988). Under healthy conditions, the normal oxygen consumption of the respiratory muscles is less than 2 percent of the total body oxygen consumption (a value approximately 5 mL/min or less), but in circumstances of extreme stress, it can increase dramatically to values approaching 125 mL/min (Field 1982). Increases in Ti/Ttot decrease the relaxation time of the diaphragm and consequently reduce diaphragmatic blood flow (Mador 1991). Measurements of $V\dot{}O_2$ respiratory muscles and values obtained in various subject and patient populations are depicted in the following Table 10.1 (Robertson 1977; Donohue 1989).

Table 10.1 Oxygen Cost of Breathing ($\dot{V}O_2$ Respiratory Muscles) (Robertson 1977; Donohue 1989)

	Absolute Values mLO$_2$/L ventilation	Percentage Total Body VO$_2$
Healthy controls	1.23 +/− 0.51	3.96 +/− 1.61%
COPD nourished	2.61 +/− 1.07	12.28 +/− 3.3%
COPD malnourished	4.28 +/− 0.98	20.95 +/− 5.21%
COPD general	8.7 +/− 9.9	24.0%

Regardless of the mechanism or cause of inspiratory muscle fatigue, the clinical result is a similar breathing pattern—that is, rapid, shallow breathing, which pattern in clinical practice is termed the rapid, shallow breathing index (RSBI). The RSBI, defined as RR (breaths/minute)/Vt (measured in liters), has been shown to assist in assessing clinical weanabilty for ICU patients in whom liberation from mechanical ventilation is being considered. In general, a RSBI greater than 105 is an accurate predictor of failure to successfully wean and extubate (Yang 1991).

Patients with severe COPD, especially during periods of acute exacerbations or at times of invasive mechanical ventilation, clearly exemplify these principles. Patients with severe COPD, given the systemic complications associated with this chronic disease, both because of overall skeletal muscle dysfunction, including the diaphragm, plus the marked degrees of hyperinflation, which reduce the pressure-generating capacity of the diaphragm by altering the ideal length-tension relationship, are set up for fatigue and subsequent respiratory failure at times of increased mechanical loads as occurs with acute exacerbation of COPD (AECOPD). Studies have shown, even in stable COPD patients, reduced muscle-generating capacity with Pgimax, Pplmax, and Pdimax values of 25 percent, 62 percent, and 49 percent of normal control values, respectively, compared to nondiseased, healthy volunteers (Marin 1999). In a group of intubated COPD patients who failed weaning, reductions in both Pdi and Pdimax were observed with the resultant ratio of these two values above the 40 percent fatiguing threshold in comparison to patients who were successfully liberated from mechanical ventilation: Pdi (cmH_2O) = 12.6 +/- 5.8 versus 15.8 +/- 3.36; Pdimax (cmH_2O) = 34.2 +/- 24.1 versus 50.5 +/- 16.1; Pdi/Pdimax = 0.456 +/- 0.08 versus 0.330 +/- 0.09 respectively, shown in Table 10.2 (Pourriat 1986). Of note, both groups of COPD patients have similar indices of central respiratory drive, thus reinforcing the fact that muscle function—and not CNS respiratory drive suppression—is the predominate mechanism of weaning failure; that is, P0.1 (cmH_2O) = 8.21 +/- 4.4 versus 6.22 +/- 2.67, respectively. Of interest, patients with asthma are exposed to airway obstruction and hyperinflation only intermittently, unlike patients with COPD, whereby the inspiratory load is constant, yet similar muscle-related physiological principles apply.

Table 10.2: Diaphragm Muscle Measurements in Patients with COPD—Comparison of Successful Liberation from Mechanical Ventilation (Pourriat 1986)

	Pdi (cmH$_2$O)	Pdimax (cmH$_2$O)	Pdi/Pdimax
Failure to wean	12.6 +/− 5.8	34.2 +/− 24.1	0.46 +/− 0.08
Success to wean	15.8 +/− 3.4	50.5 +/− 16.1	0.33 +/− 0.09

In addition to specific neuromuscular diseases and comorbid conditions that can contribute to overall total body muscle weakness and/or fatigue, especially in relation to the diaphragm, evidence suggests that mechanical ventilation can also directly contribute to decreased force-generating capacity of the diaphragm and perhaps, under certain clinical conditions, actually cause diaphragm muscle atrophy and injury. This detrimental effect would relate to not only the maximal force-generating capacity of the diaphragm but, even more importantly, endurance also. Physiological data have shown that this "disuse" diaphragmatic dysfunction occurs directly at the level of the muscle itself, and histological and biochemical data support abnormalities in myocyte and myofibrillar protein degradation and proteolysis as this basic mechanism. In a classic study evaluating structural, histological, and biochemical characteristics of diaphragm muscle biopsies obtained from fourteen brain-dead organ donors, in comparison to eight control patients, the donor specimens demonstrated (a) significant reductions in mean cross-sectional areas of both slow-twitch and fast-twitch muscle fibers: 2,025 +/− 745 µm^2 and 1,871 +/− 589 µm^2 vs. 4,725 +/− 1,547 and 3,949 +/− 1,805, representing 57 percent and 53 percent decreases in overall cross-sectional areas in association with (b) increases in active caspase-3 enzymatic activity to suggest increased proteolytic-specific diaphragmatic muscle breakdown and proteolysis of muscle protein released from the myofibrillar lattice and subsequently targeted for ubiquitin-proteasome pathway (UPP) intracellular degradation (Levine 2008; Levine 2011). A follow-up study from this same group and others confirmed these results and also expanded support for the mechanism of UPP proteolytic diaphragm-muscle-specific degradation (Hooijman 2015). These abnormalities were observed over a relatively short period of eighteen to sixty-nine hours. The therapeutic corollary of acknowledging the condition of "disuse" atrophy or damage is that the maintenance of spontaneous diaphragmatic contraction during mechanical ventilation should be beneficial in ameliorating or even preventing this ventilator-induced reduced diaphragm muscle force-generating capacity (train but do not "s-train" the respiratory muscles) but not to levels that could precipitate overuse fatigue.

References

Altose, M. D. 1988. "Pulmonary Mechanics." In *Fishman's Pulmonary Disease and Disorders*, edited by A. P. Fishman. New York: McGraw-Hill, Health Professions Division. 147–162.

American Thoracic Society / European Respiratory Society. 1999. "Skeletal Muscle Dysfunction in Chronic Obstructive Pulmonary Disease." *American Journal of Respiratory and Critical Care Medicine* 159: S1–S40.

Bellemare, F., and A. Grassino. 1982. "Effect of Pressure and Timing of Contraction of Human Diaphragm Fatigue." *American Journal of Physiology: Respiratory Environmental and Exercise Physiology* 53 (5): 1190–1195.

Cinnella, G., G. Conti, F. Lofaso, H. Lorino, A. Harf, F. Lemaire, and L. Brochard. 1996. "Effects of Assisted Ventilation on Breathing: Volume-Controlled Pressure-Controlled Ventilation." *American Journal of Respiratory and Critical Care Medicine* 153 (3): 1025–1033.

Collett, P. W., C. Roussos, P. T. Macklem. 1988. "Respiratory Mechanics." In *Textbook of Respiratory Medicine*, edited by J. F. Murray and J. A. Nadel. Philadelphia: W. B. Saunders Company. 85–128.

Decramer, M. 1988. "The Respiratory Muscles." In *Fishman's Pulmonary Disease and Disorders*, edited by A. P. Fishman. New York: McGraw-Hill, Health Professions Division. 63–71.

Donohue, M., R. M. Rogers, D. O. Wilson, and B. E. Pennock. 1989. "Oxygen Consumption of the Respiratory Muscles in Normal and in Malnourished Patients with Chronic Obstructive Lung Disease." *American Review of Respiratory Disease* 140: 385–391.

Field, S., S. M. Kelly, and P. T. Macklem. 1982. "The Oxygen Cost of Breathing in Patients with Cardiorespiratory Disease." *American Review of Respiratory Disease* 126: 9–13.

Hooijman, P. E., A. Beishuizen, C. C. Witt, M. C. de Waard, A. R. J. Girbes, A. M. E. Spoelstra-de Man, H. W. M. Niessen, et al. 2015. "Diaphragm Muscle Fiber Weakness and Ubiquitin-Proteasome Activation in Critically Ill Patients." *American Journal of Respiratory and Critical Care Medicine* 191 (10): 1126–1138.

Kelsen, S. G., and G. J. Criner. 1988. "Pump Failure: The Pathogenesis of Hypercapnic Respiratory Failure in Patients with Lung and Chest Wall Disease." In *Fishman's Pulmonary Disease and Disorders*, edited by A. P. Fishman. New York: McGraw-Hill, Health Professions Division. 2605–2625.

Levine, S., T. Nguyen, N. Taylor, M. E. Friscia, M. T. Budak, P. Rothenberg, J. Zhu, R. Sachdeva, S. Sonnad, L. R. Kaiser, N. A. Rubinstein, S. K. Powers, and J. B. Shrager. 2008. "Rapid Disuse Atrophy of Diaphragm

Fibers in Mechanically Ventilated Humans." *New England Journal of Medicine* 358: 1327–1335.

Levine, S., C. Biswas, J. Dierov, R. Barsotti, J. B. Shrager, T. Nguyen, S. Sonnad, J. C. Kucharchzuk, L. R. Kaiser, S. Singhal, and M. T. Budak. 2011. "Increased Proteolysis, Myosin Depletion, and Atrophic AKT-FOXO Signaling in Human Diaphragm Disuse." *American Journal of Respiratory and Critical Care Medicine* 183: 483–490.

Mador, M. J. 1991. "Respiratory Muscle Fatigue and Breathing Pattern." *Chest* 100: 1430–1435.

Marin, J. M., M. Montes de Oca, J. Rassulo, and B. R. Celli. 1999. "Ventilatory Drive at Rest and Perception of Exertional Dyspnea in Severe COPD." *Chest* 115: 1293–1300.

Polkey, M. I., and J. Moxham. 2001. "Clinical Aspects of Respiratory Muscle Dysfunction in the Critically Ill." *Chest* 119: 926–939.

Pourriat, J. L., Ch. Lamberto, P. H. Hoang, J. L. Fournier, and B. Vasseur. 1986. "Diaphragmatic Fatigue and Breathing Pattern during Weaning from Mechanical Ventilation in COPD Patients." *Chest* 90 (5): 703–707.

Aubier, M., C. France, R. B. Banzett, F. Bellemare, N. T. Braun, N. S. Cherniak, T. L. Clanton, et al. 1990. Report of the Respiratory Muscle Fatigue Workshop Group. "Respiratory Muscle Fatigue." *American Review of Respiratory Disease* 142: 474–480.

Robertson, C. H., G. H. Foster, and R. L. Johnson. 1977. "The Relationship of Respiratory Failure to the Oxygen Consumption of, Lactate Production by, and Distribution of Blood Flow among Respiratory

Muscles during Increasing Inspiratory Resistance." *Journal of Clinical Investigation* 59: 31–42.

Roussos, C. S., and P. T. Macklem. 1977. "Diaphragmatic Fatigue in Man." *Journal of Applied Physiology* 43 (2): 189–197.

Yang, K. L., and M. J. Tobin. 1991. "A Prospective Study of Indexes Predicting the Outcome of Trials of Weaning from Mechanical Ventilation." *New England Journal of Medicine* 324: 1445–1450.

CHAPTER 11

Abnormalities of the Chest Wall

• • •

Some representative examples of abnormal respiratory physiology for common representative diseases frequently seen in the practice of critical-care medicine will assist in understanding prior physiological principles and also in understanding abnormal physiology in specific disease states, bearing in mind the following definitions of ventilation/perfusion (V/Q) abnormalities based upon multiple inert gas elimination technique (MIGET) criteria: shunt physiology, represented by V/Q < 0.005; low V/Q, represented by 0.005 < V/Q < 0.1; high V/Q, represented by 10 < V/Q < 100; and dead space physiology, represented by V/Q > 100.

Expansion of the intrathoracic space is not uniform in that the thoracic cage expands largely anteriorly and is relatively fixed at the spine (i.e., pump-handle movement analogy) (Bergofsky 1995). There are numerous disease processes that can result in structural and anatomic abnormalities and subsequent dysfunction, dys-synchrony, or dyscoordination of the normal coordinated mechanical coupling and function of the chest wall and their resultant deleterious effects upon ventilation. However, in relation to the intensivist and critical-care physician, the two most common musculoskeletal deformities of the chest that result in both chronic respiratory insufficiency and acute respiratory failure are severe kyphoscoliosis (KS) and flail chest (chapter 17). Both musculoskeletal abnormalities cause uncoupling of the coordinated actions of the various components of the chest wall, often resulting in paradoxical movements and frequently causing the skeletal muscles, including the diaphragm, to shorten (below the ideal length-tension relationship), causing secondary muscle weakness.

Abnormal respiratory mechanics in kyphoscoliosis

Kyphoscoliosis (KS) is a disease of the spine and its articulations, resulting in spinal buckling (Bergofsky 1959). The deformity of the spine in this disorder characteristically consists of lateral displacement of spinal curvature (scoliosis) and vertebral anterioposterior angulation (kyphosis) or both. The predominate curvature is a right major thoracic curvature extending from T4–6 to TD11–L1, resulting in the "typical" curvature of deformity (Cooper 1984). For unexplained reasons, right-sided scoliosis constitutes 75–80 percent of the total spinal deformity (Bergofsky 1959). Multiple studies predominately in noncritically ill patients with KS and patients with KS undergoing orthopedic spinal/vertebral surgical corrective or stabilization procedures have shown three consistent mechanical and muscular pulmonary physiological abnormalities: (a) decreased chest-wall compliance (Ccw) or its inverse, increased chest-wall elastance (Ecw); (b) decreased lung compliance (Clung) or its inverse, increased lung elastance (Elung); and (c) respiratory muscle weakness. In addition, the severity of these physiological abnormalities was directly correlated with the magnitude of spinal deformity most commonly assessed by Cobb's angle. The magnitude of reductions in total respiratory compliance (C, rs, tot), Ccw, and Clung are inversely proportional to Cobb's angle with more devastating abnormalities dependent upon the magnitude of deformity (Kafer 1975, Figure 5; Rochester 1988; McCool 1998, Figure 97-2).

In general, patients with KS but minimal deformity as assessed by Cobb's angle (less than 50 degrees) have barely perceptible effects in lowering Ccw to measured values of 136 mL/cmH$_2$O (compared to normal healthy values approximately 200 mL/cmH$_2$O), but as Cobb's angle increases above 100 degrees, Ccw may decline to as low as 31 mL/cmH$_2$O. In fact, equations have been derived relating the abnormally reduced Ccw to the angle of Cobb with an angle deformity of 120 degrees predicting Ccw values approximately 70 mL/cmH$_2$O and more severe angles approximating 150 degrees, causing approximate reductions in Ccw near 35 mL/cmH$_2$O (Bergofsky 1995; McCool 1998). In addition, the subsequent disruption of normal mechanicothoracic coordination causes consistent reductions in virtually all lung volume measurements, causing KS patients to ventilate at rest on the relatively lower portion of the standard pressure-volume (P-V) curve with the bulk of tidal volume expansion now occurring during the relatively flat and hypocompliant portion of this curve with studies showing an absence of the normal "steep hypercompliant" S-shaped curve characteristics (Cooper 1984, Figure 6).

Table 11.1: Representative Values of Compliance (Total Respiratory, Lung, Chest Wall) in Health and Disease (Kyphoscoliosis [KS])

	Ctot, rs	Clung	Ccw
	mL/cmH$_2$O	mL/cmH$_2$O	mL/cmH$_2$O
Normal (Bergofsky 1959)	111.5	193.8	289
	(98–120)	(138–280)	(216–363)
KS subjects (Bergofsky 1959)	39.9	94.1	76.3
	(20–79)	(54–138)	(50–75)
KS subjects (Kafer 1975)	48 +/– 25	177 +/– 11	80 +/– 12
Normal (Cooper 1984)	151 +/– 56		
KS subjects (Cooper 1984)	96 +/– 13		

Similarly in a population of patients with KS, elastance measurements (Ers, tot; Elung; Ecw) were also shown to be significantly increased above normal reference values (Ers, tot = 10 cmH$_2$O/L; Elung =

5 cmH$_2$O/L; Ecw = 5 cmH$_2$O/L) as shown in the accompanying Table 11.2. (Baydur 1990).

Table 11.2: Representative Values of Elastance (Total Respiratory, Lung, Chest Wall) in Patients with Kyphoscoliosis [KS] (Baydur 1990)

	Ers, tot	Elung	Ecw
	cmH$_2$O/L	cmH$_2$O/L	cmH$_2$O/L
KS subjects	33.9 +/– 6.6	19.8 +/– 5.5	5.34 +/– 4.10
KS subjects	37.4 +/– 9.4	24.7 +/– 9.5	8.18 +/– 2.26

Although some studies have demonstrated relatively normal airflow and airway resistance parameters, some cases of significant increases in Raw have been observed, but not universally in all KS patients. Raw, inspiratory (cmH$_2$O/L/sec) = 5.34 +/– 4.10 and 8.18 +/– 2.26 (normal values = 1.39) (Baydur, 1990).

The combination of all these abnormal physiological effects creates risk factors for increased oxygen cost of breathing, at times approximately five times above normal. In a small subset of patients with severe KS, the oxygen cost of breathing ranged from 4.1 to 11.0 mLO$_2$/L (normal values for oxygen cost of breathing = 0.25–0.5 mLO$_2$/L) (Bergofsky 1959). This increased WOB was attributable to the inordinate amount of work required in moving the chest bellows; whereby WOB in KS in moving chest bellows accounted for 20–50 percent of the total WOB compared to only 18–20 percent in normal subjects (Bergofsky 1959).

ABNORMAL GAS EXCHANGE IN KYPHOSCOLIOSIS

Despite significant aberrations in lung and chest-wall mechanics, gas exchange, especially oxygenation, tends to be preserved in KS, given the absence of intrinsic lung disease per se (Bergofsky 1959). In KS patients without hypercapnia, the alveolar to arterial oxygen gradient/difference (AaO$_2$D) tends to remain normal or, if anything, only mildly elevated to approximately 14 mm Hg (Bergofsky 1959). Even as mechanical ventilatory function worsens and even in presence of arterial hypercapnia the A-a O_2 gradient still remains, either normal or again only mildly elevated with values between 14.9 mmHg and 25 mmHg (Bergofsky 1959; Kafer 1976).

Physiologically from a gas exchange perspective, the onset, development, and progression of hypercapnia is predominately related to decreases in both tidal volume (Vt) and decreased overall minute ventilation (V̇e) with preservation of relatively normal values for total pulmonary dead space. Even with marked elevations in PaCO2, Vd/Vt remains less than 40 percent ($PaCO_2$ = 38mmHg and Vd/Vt = 27%; $PaCO_2$ = 45mmHg and Vd/Vt = 32%; $PaCO_2$ = 60mmHg and Vd/Vt = 38%) (Bergofsky 1959). In contrast to the increased Vd/Vt in patients with emphysema related to loss of alveolar gas-exchange surface area and resultant overaeration of alveoli insufficiently perfused with blood, the relatively mild to modest increases in Vd/Vt in patients with KS tend to be a reflection of their overall reduced vital capacity (VC) and thus a greater relative proportion of anatomic dead space compromising tidal volume (Vt) in relation to each individual breath. In a large group of patients with KS, Vt measured 360 +/– 114 mL and Vd/Vt 43 +/– 7 percent (with range 30–54%) (Kafer 1975; Kafer 1976, Figure 3).

References

Baydur, A., S. M. Swank, C. M. Stiles, and C. S. H. Sassoon. 1990. "Respiratory Mechanics in Anesthetized Young Patients with Kyphoscoliosis." *Chest* 97: 1157–1164.

Bergofsky, E. H. 1995. "Thoracic Deformities." In *Lung Biology in Health and Disease: The Thorax Volume 85*, edited by C. Roussos. New York: Marcel-Dekker, Inc. 1915–1949.

Bergofsky, E. H., G. M. Turino, and A. P. Fishman. 1959. "Cardiorespiratory Failure in Kyphoscoliosis." *Medicine* 38: 263–318.

Cooper, D. M., J. Velasquez Rojas, R. B. Mellins, H. A. Keim, and A. L. Mansell. 1984. "Respiratory Mechanics in Adolescents with Idiopathic Scoliosis." *American Review of Respiratory Disease* 130: 16–22.

Kafer, E. 1976. "Idiopathic Scoliosis: Gas Exchange and the Age Dependence of Arterial Blood Gases." *Journal of Clinical Investigation* 58: 825–833.

Kafer, E. R. 1975. "Idiopathic Scoliosis: Mechanical Properties of the Respiratory System and the Ventilator Response to Carbon Dioxide." *Journal of Clinical Investigation* 55: 1153–1163.

McCool, F. D., and D. F. Rochester. 1998. "Nonmuscular Diseases of the Chest Wall." In *Fishman's Pulmonary Diseases and Disorders*, edited by J. A. Elias. New York: McGraw-Hill, Health Professions Division. 1541–1560.

Rochester, D. F., and L. J. Findley. 1988. "The Lungs and Neuromuscular and Chest Wall Diseases." In *Textbook of Respiratory Medicine*, edited by J. F. Murray and J. A. Nadel. Philadelphia: W. B. Saunders Company. 1942–1972.

CHAPTER 12

Pleural Effusion/ Pneumothorax/Ascites

• • •

PLEURAL EFFUSION

FEW STUDIES HAVE ACTUALLY ACCURATELY defined the volume, cellular, and chemical characteristics of "normal" pleural fluid in healthy patients without disease. One study meticulously measured the volume of pleural fluid in the right hemithorax of nonlung disease patients undergoing thoroscopic treatment for severe essential hyperhidrosis. This study of thirty-four consecutive patients measured a pleural fluid volume equal to 8.4 +/− 4.3 mL, which, when expressed per kilogram of body mass, measured 0.26 +/− 0.1 mL/kg (Noppen 2000). The developments of both transudative and exudative pleural effusions are common in critically ill patients, many of whom require invasive mechanical ventilation. Frequently, however, it is the underlying airway or parenchymal lung disease that has a much greater impact upon clinical course than the associated effusion per se. Nevertheless, an understanding of the physiological effects of pleural effusion both upon gas exchange and lung mechanics is important, especially when consideration is being undertaken in relation to the possible performance of thoracentesis and pleural-fluid drainage as a therapeutic intervention. Even though it is common perception that relief of pleural effusions when unilateral does indeed alleviate the sensation of dyspnea, the physiological correlates of this almost immediate and often dramatic clinical benefit have not always patterned the symptomatic improvement of dyspnea (Estenne 1983).

Abnormal Gas Exchange in Pleural Effusion

Most studies have demonstrated a mild degree of hypoxemia related to unilateral pleural effusions but normal values for $PaCO_2$. The benefits of large-volume thoracentesis in improving PaO_2 have been variable, with some studies showing mild improvement, others no improvement, and some even worsening in this variable. In one relatively large study, the increase in PaO_2 following thoracentesis, although significant, increased only 8 mmHg from mean prethoracentesis values of 65.7 +/- 9.6 mmHg to 73.2 +/- 11.3 mmHg (Wang 1995). However, as commonly noted, all patients experienced symptomatic relief from their dyspnea. Following therapeutic thoracentesis, one study using multiple inert gas elimination technique (MIGET) demonstrated a mild degree of intrapulmonary shunt (6.9 +/- 6.7% of cardiac output) and an increased V/Q dispersion without any diffusion limitation as the predominate cause of hypoxemia in their cohort of patients—but again noting that PaO_2 did not increase following thoracentesis 82 +/- 10 mmHg versus 83 +/- 9 mmHg (Agusti 1997). In keeping with observations of normal $PaCO_2$, the Vd/Vt fraction remained in the normal range of 27 +/- 12 percent. The authors speculated that the lack of improvement in PaO_2 was related to delay in expansion of the compressed underlying lung parenchyma.

Abnormal Respiratory Mechanics in Pleural Effusion

In experimental animal studies, three distinct pathophysiological mechanisms appear to contribute to the abnormal lung mechanics associated with unilateral pleural effusions with the latter perhaps the most significant in contributing to the sensation of dyspnea and the frequent relief of this subjective symptom following thoracentesis when most lung-specific physiological measurements fail to substantially improve. These abnormalities include pleural-pressure induced (a) lung deflation/compression, (b) outward-directed expansion of the chest wall, and (c) caudal displacement of the diaphragm (DeTroyer 2012). This latter finding is of most significance because as the diaphragm descends, its muscle fibers shorten and thus reduce the capacity of the contracting diaphragm to generate increased levels of pressure. This experimental finding would appear to be supported by clinical observations, and the suggestion that the almost immediate relief of the sense of dyspnea following thoracentesis results primarily from allowing the diaphragm to operate at its normal and more mechanically advantageous length-tension relationship (Spyratos 2007). In a study performed upon individuals receiving mechanical ventilation and using standard physiological practices to measure the various components of the work of breathing (WOB), along with compliance and resistance, when patients underwent large-volume unilateral thoracentesis, the only observed physiological variable that improved was the reduction in ventilator-induced WOB (WOBv) (Doelken 2006, Figure 4). As these patients represented a group with substantial underlying lung disease, the WOBv before thoracentesis was already significantly elevated above normal values (3.42 +/− 0.35 J/L) but did indeed improve after the therapy (2.99 +/− 0.27 J/L) (Doelken 2006).

Standard pulmonary function tests tend to show a restrictive ventilator impairment associated with reductions in total lung capacity (TLC) and forced vital capacity (FVC). In addition, measurements of static pulmonary compliance also demonstrated significant reductions with mean values equal to 0.117 +/− 0.018 L/cmH$_2$O (range 0.070–0.512) (Estenne 1983); these values correspond to an average reduction in compliance values to 38.5 percent predicted (range 18–66%) (Estenne 1983). In this particular study, similar to previous publications, following thoracentesis, there was marked improvement in relief of the sensation of dyspnea but only minor and clinically insignificant improvement in pulmonary compliance of only an average 0.021 L/cmH$_2$O, thus again reinforcing the improvement in diaphragm muscle length-tension relationship and force-generating capacity as the potential predominant mechanism for reduced symptoms.

Pneumothorax

Interpretation of the effects of either pleural effusion or pneumothorax upon lung mechanics will almost always especially in critically ill patients be complicated by the presence of underlying airway and parenchymal lung disease, thus making it difficult to accurately gauge or partition the direct effects of pleural disease abnormalities by themselves in the pure state. "Pneumothorax" (Pntx) is defined as the presence of air/gas in the pleural space. Similar to any space-occupying lesions of the pleural space, Pntx shares similar physiological abnormalities as pleural effusions, including (a) lung deflation/compression, (b) outward-directed expansion of the chest wall, and (c) caudal displacement of the diaphragm. Note that during the experimental induction of air to induce Pntx in two human patients with pulmonary tuberculosis, the reductions in lung volume measurements at end expiration amounted to only 30 percent of the volume of air instilled, implying that the remainder of instilled volume resulted in outward expansion of the chest wall and caudal displacement of the diaphragm (Christie 1936). However, in the presence of Pntx, there is an additional alteration secondary to the change in the alveolar-pleural pressure gradient, which, at the resting end-expiratory volume of the lung and chest wall at FRC, generates a negative intrapleural pressure of approximately –5 cmH$_2$O related to the outward-directed recoil of the chest wall. In the presence of a Pntx, this pressure gradient/difference is reduced with a new resting balance now achieved by the lung and chest wall, at which equilibration point no further inward lung collapse will occur. In general, even a 50 percent increase in intrapleural pressure from −5 cmH$_2$O to −2.5 cmH$_2$O will cause the respiratory system to reset at a new value between 10–30 percent below the original FRC volume (Light 1988, Figure 77-1).

The main physiological abnormalities associated with Pntx are hypoxemia and reduced vital capacity (VC). In a group of twelve patients, nine of whom had no underlying lung disease, values of PaO$_2$ ranged from 50.8 to 89.3 mmHg, but note some patients had more severe reductions in PaO$_2$ to values less than 60 mmHg (Norris 1968). The main mechanism to cause these reductions in PaO$_2$ is thought to be resultant from airway closure associated with the reduced lung volumes but with preservation of perfusion resulting in increased intrapulmonary shunt fraction with the larger the estimated size of the Pntx generating more severe degrees of hypoxemia with Pntx volumes less than 25 percent, usually well tolerated with preserved oxygenation status in patients without intrinsic lung disease (Norris 1968).

Ascites

As the diaphragm and abdominal wall are considered integral parts of the overall chest-wall component of ventilation, it should appear obvious that any factor that increases intraabdominal pressures if severe enough—or, in the case of ascites, if large enough in volume—could result in abnormal respiratory-system mechanics and potentially alterations in gas exchange. In relation to the latter physiological abnormality (i.e., hypoxemia and hypercapnia), studies have proven difficult to isolate a single mechanism alone from abdominal ascites as the sole or even major contributing factor given additional negative influences from concomitant diseases upon PaCO$_2$ and PaO$_2$. This is especially confounded in relation to the disease cirrhosis, where circulatory humoral factors usually contribute to hypocapnea, and vascular circulatory derangements (hepatopulmonary syndrome) can frequently contribute to hypoxemia. Nevertheless, in cases associated with large-volume ascites, mild degrees of hypoxemia are often reported (Byrd 1996; Chang 1997).

However, in relation to abnormal respiratory-systems mechanics, clear abnormalities have been demonstrated with the confirmatory improvement in these indices following therapeutic large-volume paracentesis. Most studies have consistently demonstrated a restrictive ventilatory impairment with reductions in both total lung capacity (TLC) and vital capacity (VC) but surprisingly usually only mild in severity with VC values recorded as 63.1 +/− 14.4 percent predicted, 65.2 +/− 14.2 percent predicted, 64 percent predicted, and 68.5 +/− 13.5 percent predicted (Abelmann 1948; Chao 1994; Byrd 1996; Chang 1997). Mechanically the instillation of fluid into the peritoneal cavity of experimental animals or from clinical observations in humans causes cranial displacement of the diaphragm with outward bulging of the abdominal muscles being observed in association with increases in intraabdominal hydrostatic pressure (Pih). These abnormalities then cause an increase in the elastance of the abdominal component of overall respiratory-system elastance and also reductions in the diaphragm's force-generating capacity (Abelmann 1954; Leduc 2009). Interestingly, it is the magnitude of increase in Pih rather than abdominal girth or height that is the most important contributing factor to these abnormal parameters, with an inverse correlation between measured VC and Pih (Hanson 1990).

Finally, similar to so many physiological processes, there also appears to be a threshold or critical volume of ascites accumulation before these mechanical physiological abnormalities become manifest, but once overt, even relatively small increases further in ascites volume will result in dramatic increases in abdominal wall elastance (Leduc 2007). In an experimental animal model, abnormal elevations in abdominal wall elastance were not evident until an instilled volume of 50 mL/kg but then rose exponentially as the instilled volume was further increased to 200 mL/kg (Leduc 2007, Figure 1). In addition, this same study also demonstrated reduced efficiency of diaphragm muscle shortening at the larger volumes of ascites.

References

Abelmann, W. H., N. R. Frank, E. A. Gaensler, and D. W. Cugell. 1954. "Effects of Abdominal Distention by Ascites on Lung Volumes and Ventilation." *Archives of Internal Medicine* 95: 528–540.

Agusti, A. G. N., J. Cardus, J. Roca, J. M. Grau, A. Xaubet, and R. Rodriguez-Roisin. 1997. "Ventilation Perfusion Mismatch in Patients with Pleural Effusions." *American Journal of Respiratory and Critical Care Medicine* 156: 1205–1209.

Byrd, R. P., T. M. Roy, and M. Simmons. 1996. "Improvement in Oxygenation after Large Volume Paracentesis." *Southern Medical Journal* 89 (7): 689–692.

Chang, S-C., H-I. Chang, F-J. Chen, G-M. Shiao, S-S. Wang, and S-D. Lee. 1997. "Therapeutic Effects of Diuretics and Paracentesis on Lung Function in Patients with Non-alcoholic Cirrhosis and Tense Ascites." *Journal of Hepatology* 26: 833–838.

Chao, Y., S-S. Wang, S-D. Lee, G-M. Shiao, H-I. Chang, and S-C. Chang. 1994. "Effect of Large Volume Paracentesis on Pulmonary Function in Patients with Cirrhosis and Tense Ascites." *Journal of Hepatology* 20: 101–105.

Christie, R. V., and C. A. McIntosh. 1936. "The Lung Volume and Respiratory Exchange after Pneumothorax." *Quarterly Journal of Medicine* 5: 445–454.

De Troyer, A., D. Leduc, M. Cappello, and P. A. Gevenois. 2012. "Mechanics of the Canine Diaphragm in Pleural Effusion." *Journal of Applied Physiology* 113: 785–790.

Doelken, P., R. Abreu, S. A. Sahn, P. H. Mayo. 2006. "Effect of Thoracentesis on Respiratory Mechanics and Gas Exchange in Patients Receiving Mechanical Ventilation." *Chest* 130: 1354–1361.

Estenne, M., J.C. Yernault, A. De Troyer. 1983. "Mechanism of Relief of Dyspnea after Thoracentesis in Patients with Large Pleural Effusions." *American Journal of Medicine* 74 (5): 813–819.

Hanson, C. A., A. B. Ritter, W. Duran, and M. H. Lavietes. 1990. "Ascites: Its Effect upon Static Inflation of the Respiratory System." *American Review of Respiratory Disease* 142: 39–42.

Leduc, D., and A. De Troyer. 2007. "Dysfunction of the Canine Respiratory Muscle Pump in Ascites." *Journal of Applied Physiology* 102: 650–657.

Leduc, D., and A. De Troyer. 2009. "Mechanism of Increased Inspiratory Rib Elevation in Ascites." *Journal of Applied Physiology* 107: 734–740.

Light, R. W. 1988. "Pneumothorax." In *Textbook of Respiratory Medicine*, edited by J. F. Murray and J. A. Nadel. Philadelphia: W. B. Saunders Company. 1745–1759.

Noppen, M., M. De Waele, R. Li, K. Vander Gucht, J. D'Haese, E. Gerlo, and W. Vincken. 2000. "Volume and Cellular Content of Normal Pleural Fluid in Humans Examined by Pleural Lavage." *American Journal of Respiratory and Critical Care Medicine* 162: 1023–1026.

Norris, R. M., J. G. Jones, and J. M. Bishop. 1968. "Respiratory Gas Exchange in Patients with Spontaneous Pneumothorax." *Thorax* 23: 427–433.

Spyratos, D., L. Sichletidis, K. Manika, T. Kontakiotis, D. Chloros, and D. Patakas. 2007. "Expiratory Flow Limitation in Patients with Pleural Effusions." *Interventional Pulmonology* 74: 572–578.

Wang, J-S., and C. H. Tseng. 1995. "Changes in Pulmonary Mechanics and Gas Exchange after Thoracentesis on Patients with Inversion of a Hemi-Diaphragm Secondary to Large Pleural Effusion." *Chest* 107: 1610–1614.

CHAPTER 13
Venous-Thromboembolic Disease

• • •

PULMONARY EMBOLISM (PE) AND DEEP venous thrombosis (DVT) represent the spectrum of one disease, termed venous-thromboembolic disease (VTE). Approximately 80 percent of patients presenting with PE will have evidence of DVT in their lower extremities. Conversely, pulmonary embolism occurs in up to 50 percent of patients with proximal DVT (Tapson 2008). In the United States, the incidence of PE approximates one episode for every thousand patients with estimated annual frequency of greater than six hundred thousand patients. In addition, estimates project an annual death rate directly attributable to PE between fifty thousand and three hundred thousand (Wood 2002; Tapson 2008). Many such deaths occur suddenly with diagnosis of PE only being confirmed at autopsy. A subpopulation of patients defined as having major or massive PE frequently require emergent care in the ICU setting. These patients are often defined based upon echocardiographic findings of right-ventricle dysfunction but more commonly based upon clinical presentation of hemodynamic instability, shock, cardiac and circulatory arrest, or refractory hypoxemia. Variable mortality rates are reported for patients with major PE based solely upon echocardiographic findings, but clearly shock or cardiac arrest carry excessive mortality rates between 30 and 70 percent, even with appropriate clinical management (Wood 2002). Although life-threatening PE traditionally has been equated with greater than 50 percent occlusion/

obstruction of the pulmonary vascular bed, it has also become clear that not only the amount or size of pulmonary vascular occlusion (i.e., clot burden) but also the underlying cardiopulmonary status are key components in contributing to either survival or death (McIntyre 1974; Wood 2002).

Abnormal Gas Exchange in Pulmonary Embolism

As would be expected, multiple factors influence/affect the abnormal gas exchange associated with acute PE, including the magnitude of pulmonary vascular occlusion; the duration of VTE onset since diagnosis; associated parenchymal complications such as hemorrhage, atelectasis, or infarction; time frame; therapies; and, perhaps surprisingly, the hemodynamic or cardiac output response to the acute pulmonary vascular occlusion and resultant increase in pulmonary vascular resistance (PVR). Using the multiple inert gas elimination technique (MIGET), various patterns and mechanisms of abnormal gas exchange have been identified, which can vary from patient to patient for the prior noted reasons but which usually result in the same endpoints—namely, hypoxemia, hypocapnia, and increased minute ventilation ($\dot{V}e$). Using the previously noted MIGET definitions, it has been demonstrated that in early stages of acute PE, the mechanism of hypoxemia is dominated by regions of low V/Q, but in association with the later development of parenchymal infiltrates (hemorrhage, infarction, atelectasis), small levels of anatomic shunt, usually less than 5 percent, also become contributing factors—but only in the presence of preserved cardiac output (CO) and the absence of shock (West 1991, Figure 13; Santolicandro 1995).

The anatomic mechanism contributing to these areas of low V/Q is actually quite simplistic. In the presence of pulmonary vascular occlusion, the body's response is to still maintain "normal" levels of cardiac output and systemic tissue perfusion to meet overall total body metabolic needs which, in effect, increases flow (Q) to areas of non-embolic occluded alveoli with preserved (not exaggerated) ventilation, thus causing V/Q to drop due to an increase in the denominator (Q) without a compensatory increase in the numerator (V) (Huet 1985). Hypoxemia occurs as a consequence of vascular occlusion when increased or preserved cardiac output is redistributed from obstructed to nonobstructed vessels (Manier 1992). As long as cardiac output is maintained, this results in an overall overperfusion of areas of nonoccluded lung segments, reducing V/Q and contributing to hypoxemia. This becomes even more exaggerated in situations of reduced ventilation such as infarcted or atelectatic areas of lung resulting in an almost true anatomic shunt physiology.

In addition, it should be obvious that in diseased areas of vascular occluded lung without associated hemorrhage, infarction, atelectasis, these "abnormal" areas of perfusion with "normal" ventilation will then exceed perfusion resulting in increased V/Q ratios in the direction of worsening dead-space ventilation as another common finding in acute PE (Elliott 1992). However, in general, the degree of dead-space elevation, usually 40–60 percent, is nowhere near the magnitude associated with severe obstructive airway disease, and the central nervous system (CNS) stimulus for increased minute ventilation is more than capable of overriding the worsening dead-space ventilation to result actually in the common observation of acute respiratory alkalosis and reduced $PaCO_2$ rather than hypercapnia.

However, in the presence of massive/major PE, usually associated with the abrupt occlusion of 40–50 percent of the pulmonary vascular bed or in association with prior concomitant cardiovascular disease, the right ventricle acutely fails and can no longer generate the pressures necessary to maintain adequate forward flow and sustained systemic tissue perfusion (reduced DO_2), resulting in increased peripheral-tissue oxygen extraction, causing marked reductions in mixed venous-oxygen tensions (MVO_2) and saturations, often to levels less than 30 mmHg and 50 percent hemoglobin saturation. This marked drop in oxygen content returning from the venous circulation to the right side of the heart, then in association with existent areas of low V/Q for the above noted reasons, becomes the driving force for greater degrees of hypoxemia. The improvement in oxygenation might then be considered an indicator of improved cardiac output (Dantzker 1979). Similar results have been demonstrated in experimental animal models of acute PE (Tsang 2005).

In summary, the changes in V/Q relationship after acute PE are mainly the result of the dynamic redistribution of regional perfusion (Q) to nonoccluded areas of lung and, to a lesser extent, redistribution of ventilation. These lower V/Q regions created by this higher flow are then found in the less embolized regions, presumably due to vascular recruitment, as in these areas of nonoccluded pulmonary circulation, local resistance would be lowest. The hypoxemia of acute PE can then be explained by *new* low V/Q regions resulting from the local redistribution of regional perfusion without adequate compensatory increases or changes in regional ventilation (Altemeier 1998; Ferreira 2006). In situations of shock and acute right-ventricular (RV) failure, the development of low MVO_2 can significantly affect PaO_2 by decreasing end-capillary PO_2 of lung units with V/Q ratios less than one. Thus, in clinical situations of large clot burden / vascular occlusion and right-ventricular decompensation, the combination of relatively mild V/Q inequality and low MVO_2 will cause severe hypoxemia.

Finally, an additional mechanism of intractable hypoxemia also bears mention that can be observed in any situation of acute and marked elevations in PVR but has been commonly reported in PE. This mechanism includes the transient hemodynamically generated physiological opening of the foramen ovale that allows for a true anatomic right-to-left shunt through the cardiac atria, which, under normal situations, remains closed because of the usual higher pressure gradients from the left to the right heart that become reversed under conditions of acute massive PE. Perhaps of even more clinical significance than the arterial blood gas abnormalities is this same mechanism as a contributing factor to paradoxical pulmonary embolism that can have severe systemic circulation consequences, such as acute stroke or systemic arterial tissue infarction (D'Alonzo 1983; Estagnasie 1996; Rajan 2007; Moua 2008).

REFERENCES

Altemeier, W. A., H. T. Robertson, S. McKinney, and R. W. Glenny. 1998. "Pulmonary Embolization Causes Hypoxemia by Redistributing Regional Blood Flow without Changing Ventilation." *Journal of Applied Physiology* 85 (6): 2337–2343.

D'Alonzo, G. E., J. S. Bower, P. DeHart, and D. R. Dantzker. 1983. "The Mechanisms of Abnormal Gas Exchange in Acute Massive Pulmonary Embolism." *American Review of Respiratory Disease* 128: 170–172.

Dantzker, D. R., and J. S. Bower. 1979. "Mechanism of Gas Exchange Abnormalities in Patients with Chronic Obliterative Pulmonary Vascular Disease." *Journal of Clinical Investigation* 64: 1050–1055.

Elliott, G. 1992. "Pulmonary Physiology during Pulmonary Embolism." *Chest* 101 (4): 163S–171S.

Estagnasie, P., K. Djedaini, G. Le Bourdelles, F. Coste, and D. Dreyfuss. 1996. "Atrial Septal Aneurysms plus a Patent Foramen Ovale." *Chest* 110: 846–848.

Ferreira, J. H. T., R. G. G. Terzi, I. A. Paschoal, W. A. Silva, A. C. Moraes, and M. M. Moreira. 2006. "Mechanisms of Underlying Gas Exchange Alterations in an Experimental Model of Pulmonary Embolism." *Brazilian Journal of Medical and Biological Research* 39 (9): 1197–1204.

Huet, Y., F. Lemaire, C. Brun-Buisson, W. A. Knaus, B. Teisseire, D. Payen, D. Mathieu. 1985. "Hypoxemia in Acute Pulmonary Embolism." *Chest* 88 (6): 829–836.

Manier, G., and Y. Castaing. 1992. "Influence of Cardiac Output on Oxygen Exchange in Acute Pulmonary Embolism." *American Review of Respiratory Disease* 145: 130–136.

McIntyre, K. M., and A. A. Sasahara. 1974. "Determinants of Right Ventricular Function and Hemodynamics after Pulmonary Embolism." *Chest* 65 (5): 534–543.

Moua, T., K. E. Wood, B. D. Atwater, and J. R. Runo. 2008. "Major Pulmonary Embolism and Hemodynamic Stability from Shunting through a Patent Foramen Ovale." *Southern Medical Journal* 101: 955–958.

Rajan, G. R. 2007. "Intractable Intraoperative Hypoxemia Secondary to Pulmonary Embolism in the Presence of Undiagnosed Patent Foramen Ovale." *Journal of Clinical Anesthesiology* 19: 374–377.

Santolicandro, A., R. Prediletto, E. Fornai, B. Formichi, E. Beglomini, A. Giannella-Neto, and C. Giuntini. 1995. "Mechanisms of Hypoxemia and Hypocapnia in Pulmonary Embolism." *American Journal of Respiratory and Critical Care Medicine* 152: 336–347.

Tapson, V. F. 2008. "Acute Pulmonary Embolism." *New England Journal of Medicine* 358: 1037–1052.

Tsang, J. Y., W. J. E. Lamm, I. R. Starr, and M. P. Hlastala. 2005. "Spatial Pattern of Ventilation Perfusion Mismatch following Acute Pulmonary Thromboembolism in Pigs." *Journal of Applied Physiology* 98: 1862–1868.

West, J. B., and P. D. Wagner. 1991. "Ventilation Perfusion Relationships." In *The Lung Scientific Foundations*, edited by R. G. Crystal and J. B. West. New York: Raven Press. 1289–1305.

Wood, K. E. 2002. "Major Pulmonary Embolism: Review of a Pathophysiological Approach to the Golden Hour of Hemodynamically Significant Pulmonary Embolism." *Chest* 121 (3): 877–905.

CHAPTER 14

Obstructive Airways Diseases

• • •

Chronic Obstructive Pulmonary Disease

COPD IS DEFINED AS "A preventable and treatable disease state characterized by airflow limitation that is not fully reversible. The airflow limitation is usually progressive and associated with an abnormal inflammatory response of the lungs to inhaled noxious particles or gases, primarily caused by cigarette smoking. Although COPD affects the lungs, it also produces significant systemic consequences" (Celli 2004, page 933). Pathologically COPD is not a single disease but represents a combination of two unique, distinct, and anatomically site-specific disease processes, namely emphysema and chronic obstructive bronchitis. The obstructive physiology (expiratory airflow limitation) essential for the diagnosis of COPD is classically thought to result from a) emphysema-mediated tissue destruction with consequent loss of elastic recoil and reduced tethering of the airway lumen plus b) bronchiolitis-related inflammation with impingement upon the airway lumen and mucus impaction. In addition to the previously identified and established loss of alveolar capillary gas-exchange surface area because of progressive inflammatory cell mediated proteolytic destruction of alveolar walls in emphysema, it has also been recently demonstrated that in all stages of COPD disease severity there also exists a drop-out and reduction in both number and airway surface area of terminal bronchioles 2.0 to 2.5

mm diameter with more severe physiological impairment as evidenced by FEV1 measurements directly correlated with larger volumes/profusion of airway loss and reduced airway surface area (McDonough 2011). This recent data indicates the importance of structural damage to the airways of patients with COPD analogous to alveolar wall destruction in emphysema with the resultant loss of airway surface area also representing a major component to increased airway resistance and not simple bronchospasm or lumen occlusion by mucus and inflammatory debris. In non-diseased control lung specimens, the total number of terminal bronchioles equaled 22,300 +/- 3900, and the total cross sectional area was 3050.3 +/- 576.6 mm^2 per lung (McDonough 2011). Lung specimens from patients with severe COPD and centrilobular emphysema demonstrated an 89% reduction in total number of terminal bronchioles per lung and a drastic 99.7% reduction in terminal bronchiole cross sectional area (McDonough 2011).

COPD is a common disease with estimates of frequency affecting approximately 4–5 percent of the US population with an estimated prevalence of twenty to twenty-five million individuals. Although cigarette smoking is by far the major risk factor for development of COPD, occupational, environmental, and even home exposures, such as indoor cooking and heating with combustible carbon products, are being identified as significant contributing risk factors. Currently COPD is listed as the fourth-leading cause of death worldwide and is listed on one of twenty death certificates in the United States. Despite the emphasis on the chronic nature of COPD and the systemic complications, only approximately 10 percent of the entire COPD population actually dies as a result of a respiratory-related event. The vast majority of patients with COPD die as a result of smoking-induced associated cardiovascular complications or malignancies. Even focusing on the subpopulation of patients dying because of COPD, it is clearly evident that the interval development of acute respiratory events on top of severe physiological impairment from the chronic component of COPD (usually defined as FEV1 < 40% predicted) are the main determinants of fatality.

These interspersed acute events are termed acute exacerbations of COPD (AECOPD) and are defined clinically as "an acute change in a patient's baseline dyspnea, cough, and/or sputum production beyond day-to-day variability sufficient to warrant a change in therapy" (www.gold-copd.org). Approximately 750,000 hospitalizations per year occur in the United States with a diagnosis of AECOPD; even more importantly, these 750,000 yearly hospitalizations result in approximately 150,000 directly related COPD respiratory deaths (Chandra 2012). AECOPD have a major impact of patient quality of life (QOL) and morbidity in association with persistent high mortality of 3–5 percent per hospitalization and approaching 20 percent if requiring intubation and initiation of mechanical ventilation. Even for patients who survive these index hospitalizations, on average, they still manifest an approximate 50 percent mortality at five years (Soler-Cataluna 2005). These acute exacerbations are somewhat predictable and not just random occurrences, but of most importance is the fact that the more severe the baseline level of COPD lung impairment, the more frequent the occurrence of acute exacerbations; and it is this specific population of patients that requires hospitalization and frequently results in inpatient death in an intensive-care unit (ICU) or hospital setting. In addition, the most reliable predictive risk factor for the development of an AECOPD remains a prior history of an AECOPD—that is, the AECOPD phenotype of COPD, whereby AECOPD begets AECOPD. These statistics should not be surprising, as the frequency and severity of AECOPD and consequently morbidity and mortality are directly related to the severity of baseline lung function, and thus these statistics are greatly skewed to the COPD population with severe physiological impairment as assessed by FEV1 percent predicted—usually less than 40 percent. Noninvasive nasal/full-face ventilation with bilevel positive airway pressure (BiPAP) has become the mainstay of acute management of hypercapnic ($PaCO_2$ > 55 mmHg) patients presenting for emergent therapy of an AECOPD (Brochard 1995). However, even with this significant therapeutic advancement, approximately 20–30 percent of patients will "fail" BiPAP therapy and require invasive mechanical ventilation, and an approximately similar percentage will require intubation and mechanical ventilation upon immediate medical presentation (Chandra 2012).

ABNORMAL GAS EXCHANGE IN COPD

For both stable patients with COPD and COPD patients during the course of an acute exacerbation, it has clearly been established that mechanisms for both abnormal gas exchange profiles of hypoxemia and hypercapnia are mediated solely through V/Q mismatch without any evidence of diffusion impairment and without any evident increase in true shunt fraction (Wagner 1977; Marthan 1985; West 1991; Rodriguez-Roisin 2009). However, as is true for virtually all pulmonary diseases, for each individual patient, multiple other factors influence their gas exchange characteristics, including comorbid disease, reduced respiratory muscle strength and endurance, and cardiac function (Rodriguez-Roisin 2009). However, as specifically relates to the critical-care physician, the key clinical issue centers around the admission and management of hospitalized patients who are experiencing an acute exacerbation of their COPD (AECOPD). As expected in patients with severe COPD (defined as FEV1 < 40% predicted), severe aberrations in gas exchange (both hypoxemia and hypercapnia) are common, and for this class severity of patients, it has been clearly demonstrated that the administration of domiciliary supplemental oxygen to stable patients with resting hypoxemia defined as PaO_2 < 55 mmHg has demonstrated improved survival. In this stable population of symptomatic COPD patients, it again has been clearly demonstrated that the major mechanism of both hypoxemia and hypercapnia is abnormal V/Q mismatch (Wagner 1977), but the particular pattern of abnormal V/Q mismatch in each individual patient is variable and has led to the commonly utilized descriptive COPD phenotypes of the "pink puffer" (PP) and the "blue bloater" (BB) (Wagner 1977; Marthan1985; Wagner 1991; West 1991, Figure 10).

The "PP" COPD phenotype is characterized clinically by marked chest-wall hyperinflation and marked increases in lung residual volume (i.e., air trapping) but persistent and excessive ventilator drive (increased V'e) in attempts to maintain normal levels of gas exchange in the presence of significant elevations in Vd/Vt but with preservation of PaO_2. The "BB" is a descriptive COPD patient phenotype presumed dominated by the chronic bronchitis clinical phenotype/characteristics associated with hypercapnia, hypoxemia, and cor pulmonale. The "PP" V/Q mismatch results from a shift of blood flow from areas of reduced lung density (c/w emphysema) and creating high V/Q relationships resultant from alveolar capillary destruction. These high V/Q regions (increased dead space) in COPD are produced by the continued ventilation of regions of emphysematous alveolar destruction with resultant greatly reduced blood flow to these areas, causing increased Vd/Vt (dead-space fraction/ratio) and resulting hypercapnia, even in the face of increased minute ventilation (hypercapnia without hypoventilation). In patients with "BB" phenotype, the areas of low V/Q are thought to result from mucus obstruction and chronic inflammation of the peripheral airways, which maintain perfusion and thus create low V/Q shuntlike physiology and resultant hypoxemia. Of note, especially in relation to the "BB" COPD phenotype, another factor of relevance in determining PaO_2 is the mixed venous MVO_2 value, where for any degree of decreased V/Q relationship in shunt direction (i.e., venous admixture), any reduction in MVO_2 (below normal values 40 mmHg/ 75 percent saturation) will result in an obligatory further decreases in end-capillary PO_2 and thus PaO_2 (Wagner 1991).

Similar to many physiological processes, both in patients with COPD and asthma, relatively severe reductions in obstructive airways impairment (i.e., FEV1) must develop before the onset of hypercapnia (Kelsen 1998, Figure 171-16). However, once hypercapnia is overt, even relatively trivial or minor further worsening of airflow limitation will result in dramatic and exponential further increases in $PaCO_2$. Even in COPD patients in a stable state, significant elevations in Vd/Vt have been demonstrated with more severe values of dead-space fraction observed with greater degrees of arterial hypercapnia: normocapnia COPD patients with measured Vd/Vt = 48.6 +/− 7.9 percent; moderate hypercapnia Vd/

Vt = 55.2 +/– 9.0 percent; and severe hypercapnia Vd/Vt = 61.3 +/– 7.0 percent (Begin 1991).

In the clinical situation of patients presenting with severe AECOPD, usually requiring hospitalization and often intubation and invasive mechanical ventilation, these same relationships apply but are compounded by additional physiological stresses that are at times iatrogenically induced—that is, oversedation and hyperoxygenation. Virtually all patients presenting for hospitalization because of an AECOPD will have worsening hypoxemia, and preservation of oxygenation status and adequate tissue oxygen delivery continue to remain the most important aspects of respiratory management. An interesting phenomenon is the lack of significant supplemental oxygen-induced elevations of $PaCO_2$ in stable hypoxemic COPD patients who are prescribed continuous domiciliary supplemental oxygen on a long-term basis but the almost universal and at times somewhat dramatic increase in degree of hypercapnia for unstable COPD patients during the course of an acute exacerbation who are emergently administered increased concentrations of O_2 above their standard concentrations of chronic O_2 supplementation. This mechanism of hypoxemia again relates to worsening V/Q relationships; however, the administration of supplemental oxygen, although clearly indicated, can actually be quite slow to correct the hypoxemia and can commonly contribute to worsening CO_2 elimination and increased degrees of hypercapnia, sometimes to the point of significant global mental sedation, coma, and CO_2 narcosis. The reason for the sometimes slow improvement in oxygenation following supplemental oxygen administration is due to the extremely low equilibration times in distended emphysematous lung units with reduced elastic recoil, which takes prolonged times to effectively wash out residual nitrogen (N_2) concentrations by the increased concentrations of supplemental inspired O_2 (Wagner 1991).

Eldridge et al. (1968) have clearly demonstrated the instability of the ventilatory status of patients hospitalized for AECOPD and the observation that virtually all patients, when administered increasing concentrations of supplemental oxygen during this acute period, will develop worsening hypercapnia, but what is most revealing from this study is the unpredictability of the rate and magnitude of $PaCO_2$ elevation, with some patients demonstrating slowly rising curves and others abrupt increases in $PaCO_2$ to levels of CO_2 that can cause narcosis and sedation at even low levels of additional oxygen supplementation (Eldridge 1968, Figure 4; Hanson 1996). The reason for worsening hypercapnia in the setting of supplemental oxygen administration during acute therapy for AECOPD is probably twofold. The first is a mild reduction in central respiratory neurological drive due to suppression of carotid body-mediated increased ventilation resultant from hypoxemia, but this effect is usually transient within the first hours of supplemental oxygen administration and only a relatively minor contributor to increased levels of arterial $PaCO_2$ (Robinson 2000). Of even greater significance is the abrupt release of compensatory hypoxic vasoconstriction in areas of partially or poorly ventilated alveoli following the indiscriminate administration of high levels of supplemental oxygen that can actually steal perfusion (Q) from other, better-ventilated and less hypoxic alveoli. This "vascular steal" syndrome is the direct result of the release of hypoxic vasoconstriction in more severely hypoxemia and poorly ventilated lung units, which then increase perfusion to these regions but steal blood flow from other regions (Robinson 2000). The resultant net increase in $PaCO_2$ results from a relative increase in wasted dead-space (Vd/Vt) ventilation greater than the increase in minute ventilation (acknowledging reduced respiratory muscle strength, stamina, and endurance during episodes of acute exacerbations) such that the resultant effective alveolar ventilation (V̇A) actually drops, even in face of increased CO_2 production (Eldridge 1968; Dick 1997; Schumaker 2004).

Thus the increase in V/Q and consequent increase in Vd/Vt results predominantly from a decrease in the denominator (Q) from well-functioning alveolar units without a compensatory decrease in the numerator (V). As reinforcement of this concept, the similar physiological scenario for worsening hypercapnia was observed in a cohort of patients with severe but stable COPD, whereby hyperoxia (60% FiO_2) caused the release of regional hypoxic vasoconstriction with worsening of V/Q mismatch, expansion of dead-space ventilation, and reduction in efficiency of CO_2 elimination. This increase in $PaCO_2$ (11.6 +/- 2.2 mmHg) was mainly explained by the hyperoxia-induced increase in Vd/Vt as minute ventilation (V̇e), and V̇CO_2 actually fell in proportion by only a small amount (O'Donnell 2002). Previous studies using multiple inert gas elimination technique (MIGET) technology also demonstrated that when hyperoxia caused release of hypoxic vasoconstriction in previously underperfused and poorly ventilated alveolar units, blood was diverted from alveolar units with relatively preserved V/Q ratios, these latter units then becoming converted into units with high V/Q, which compensatorily increased Vd/Vt, ultimately worsening the degree of hypercapnia (Robinson 2000).

Finally, as continually noted, any episode of hypercapnic respiratory failure is always a combination of increased work of breathing and reduced respiratory muscle function, again stressing the importance of BiPAP in the setting of acute hypercapnic AECOPD whereby the most significant physiological benefit appears to be enhanced diaphragmatic function and relieving the strain upon the already compromised and fatiguing respiratory muscles and subsequent improvement in the balance between increased work of breathing (WOB) and the capacity of the respiratory muscles to compensate for this force/work overload. Again recalling the various determinant of $PaCO_2$ by the equation $PaCO_2 = 0.863 \times \dot{V}eCO_2/\dot{V}e (1 - Vd/Vt)$, often not mentioned, but again, another potential contribution to worsening hypercapnia is an increased V̇eCO_2 resultant from the marked activation of the respiratory muscles and stress of the hypercatabolic acute clinical state, which will only lead to increased needs for extra augmented ventilation in presence of an already reduced muscular sustainability and endurance.

Asthma

Asthma is a syndrome of nonspecific airway hyperresponsiveness, inflammation, and intermittent respiratory symptoms triggered by infection, environmental allergens, or other stimuli. Severe asthma is characterized by persistent symptoms, increased medication requirements, persistent airflow limitation, and frequent exacerbations. Although severe asthma is estimated to be present in less than 10 percent of all patients with asthma, these patients exhibit the greatest morbidity and consume an overwhelming proportion of healthcare costs (Wahidi 2012). Asthma is often defined as "a common chronic disorder of the airways that is complex and characterized by variable and recurring symptoms, airflow obstruction, bronchial hyperresponsiveness, and underlying inflammation" (Lotvall 2011). Although both COPD and asthma are characterized physiologically as obstructive lung diseases, their pathology, etiology, clinical course, prognosis, risk factors, and management are markedly different. This becomes even more evident in comparison of acute asthmatic exacerbations and acute COPD exacerbations in relation to mechanisms of abnormal gas exchange—namely, hypoxemia and hypercapnia.

Asthma remains a fatal disease with an estimated five hundred deaths per year, often sudden and unexpected and predominantly affecting young children, adolescents, or young adults. Asthma patients with severe disease represent the greatest unmet medical need in terms of understanding mechanisms, morbidity, healthcare costs, and effective treatment for this heterogeneous group of diseases labeled under the all-inclusive term "asthma" (Jarjour 2012). Potential identifying features for adults with severe asthma include (a) frequent use of systemic corticosteroids; (b) history of frequent hospitalizations or any single intubation; (c) increased prevalence of comorbid disease such as obesity, sinusitis, or pneumonia; (d) marked or severe airflow limitation on spirometry with incomplete reversibility; and (e) air trapping (defined as residual volume [RV] > 120% predicted) and hyperinflation (defined as total lung capacity [TLC] > 120% predicted) on pulmonary function tests (PFTs) (Moore 2007; Jarjour 2012). Patients with abrupt-onset, life-threatening asthma also appear to have both persistent structural changes in the airways and a different inflammatory cell profile compared to stable, controlled patients with asthma. These structural changes include increased thickening of both the airway epithelium and lamina reticularis (Cohen 2007; Jarjour 2012). The inflammatory cell profile frequently represents a predominance of neutrophils (polymorphonuclear leukocytes—PMNs) rather than the typical IgE allergic-atopic mediated eosinophilic inflammatory patterned response (Sur 1993; Ordonez 2000).

Abnormal gas exchange in acute status asthmaticus: Arterial hypoxemia is nearly universally present in all patients during acute asthmatic exacerbations and frequently can lag behind in recovery in comparison to the improved lung mechanics as evidenced by measurements of expiratory flow such as peak expiratory flow rate (PEFR) or forced expiratory volume in one second (FEV1) (Wagner 1978; Wagner 1987; Roca 1988; Ferrer 1993). Patients with severe asthma typically display a bimodal pattern of V/Q relationships: (a) distinct population of lung units with low V/Q ratios ($0.005 < V/Q < 0.1$) and (b) distinct population of lung units with normal V/Q ratios. True shunt is almost always absent in association also, with no evidence of diffusion impairment. In small numbers of asthma patients during acute exacerbations, true shunt values have been measured, representing 1.5 +/− 2.3 percent of all V/Q values, but much more significant are the substantial increases in perfusion of lung units with reduced V/Q values being measured at 27.6 +/− 12.3 percent (Rodriguez-Roisin 1989; West 1991, Figure 9; Rodrigo 2004).

However, in relation to mechanisms of hypercapnia, and in stark contrast to patients with COPD, there exists a virtual absence of areas of high V/Q ratio inequality causing increased dead space Vd/Vt values, accounting for only approximately 3 percent of the total requirement for increased ventilation (Rodriguez-Roisin 1989). This absence of increased dead space most surely relates to the absence of alveolar-wall destruction in asthma, for which destruction remains the hallmark pathological finding in emphysema. These observations have been reproduced in other human studies and experimental animal models also (Wagner 1978; Rubinfeld 1978). Thus the mechanism of hypoxemia between asthma and COPD may be similar, but the causation of hypercapnia and resultant ventilator failure are distinctly different, with muscular failure being the primary cause of hypercapnia in asthma—given the markedly increased work of breathing—but both muscle fatigue and, probably more importantly, markedly increased dead space ventilation are predominate contributors to severe hypercapnia during acute exacerbations of COPD. Although not often considered, fundamental differences in specific anatomic locations mediating increases in airway resistance between the small peripheral airways (less than 2 mm internal diameter) and the larger central airways probably also contribute to increased WOB evident in asthmatic patients during episodes of fatal or near-fatal acute respiratory failure (ARF), where pathological evidence or even bronchoscopic examination reveals severe large airway narrowing to luminal diameters almost negligible, marked edema, and airway swelling, with superimposed high-grade proximal airway mucus impaction, again not commonly evident in patients presenting with AECOPD, where the predominant site of disease is localized to the small peripheral terminal bronchioles.

Abnormal Respiratory Mechanics in Obstructive Airway Disease (Asthma and COPD)

The hallmark physiological abnormalities in acute asthma and acute exacerbations of COPD (AECOPD) are derived primarily from the marked increase in airway resistance (Raw), both peripheral and central, which in turn creates secondary downstream effects of air trapping, hyperinflation, and hypocompliant overdistended chest wall (McFadden 2003). However, of note, the physiological abnormalities, although severe, are often transient and intermittent in asthma and chronic, progressive, and persistent in COPD. As previously noted, for patients with asthma or COPD requiring invasive mechanical ventilation, Raw can be calculated by taking the difference between Ppeak and Pplateau divided by inspiratory flow rate; that is, $Raw = (Ppk - Pplat)/\dot{V}i$ (Tobin 1988, Figure 6; Tobin 1990, Figure 3; Ward 1994, Figure 4-43; Dhand 1995, Figure 1; Jubran 1996, Figure 9; Gattionni 2006; Singer 2009).

In COPD the pulmonary Raw can increase to 5–15 cmH$_2$O/L/sec compared to a normal value of 1–2 cmH$_2$O/L/sec (Loring 2009); and another study demonstrated mean Raw values equal to 21.1 +/– 1.0 in a cohort of patients with COPD receiving mechanical ventilation (Ranieri 1997). The marked increase in airway resistance often results in the requirement for intubation and initiation of invasive mechanical ventilation causing dramatic increases in ventilator-induced peak airway pressure with contributions both from increased Raw (nonelastic work) and hypocompliance (elastic work) of the chest wall, the latter often noted as an increase in ventilator plateau pressure, which is flow independent, with the former (increased Raw) being predominant (Leatherman 1996, Figure 1; Fernandez-Perez 2005, Figure 1).

In one study of patients with asthma receiving mechanical ventilation, average values for peak (Ppk) and plateau (Pplat) airway pressures while receiving mechanical ventilation at Vt = 12 mL/kg, RR = 14/min and inspiratory flow 80 L/min were approximately Ppk = 64 and Pplat = 25 cmH$_2$O respectively, generating Ppk – Pplat differences approximately 40 cmH$_2$O, which are well above the expected normal value near 5–10 cmH$_2$O (Tuxen 1994; Leatherman 1996).

These values physiologically reflect the predominant effect of the increased WOB attributable to overcoming Raw and less pressure to overcome the elastic properties of the lung for patients with asthma. In a study of twelve patients requiring mechanical ventilation for status asthmaticus, representative values for ventilator-induced Ppeak measured 66.8 +/– 8.7 cmH$_2$O (RR = 18); 66.4 +/– 9.5 cmH$_2$O (RR = 12); and 67.8 +/– 11/1 cmH$_2$O (RR = 6) compared to respective representative values of Pplat measuring 25.4 +/– 2.8 cmH$_2$O (RR = 18); 23.3 +/– 2.6 cmH$_2$O (RR = 12); and 21.3 +/– 2.9 cmH$_2$O (RR = 6) (Leatherman, 2004). In fact, reductions in the mechanical ventilator-induced Ppk – Pplat gradient have been implicated as evidence of reductions in Raw and improved lung mechanics in patients with severe asthma as a positive response to therapy (Dhand 1995). In this same study, substantial generations of auto-PEEP were also evident.

Table 14.1: Measured Ventilator Mechanical Parameters in a Population of Patients with COPD or Asthma and Respiratory Failure

	Ppeak (cmH$_2$O)	Pplateau (cmH$_2$O)
COPD (Dhand 1995)	39.6 (30–48)	19.4 (13–24)
COPD (Georopoulos 1993)	42.2 (32.5–61.2)	24.8 (17.2–30.8)
Asthma (Leatherman 2004)		
RR = 6	67.8 +/– 11.1	21.3 +/– 2.9
RR = 12	66.4 +/– 9.5	23.3 +/– 2.6
RR = 18	66.8 +/– 8.7	25.4 +/– 2.8

These latter values are graphically depicted in Figure 1 of the referenced citation (Leatherman 2004).

Although values for plateau pressure (Pplat) are quite similar for both groups of patients with obstructive airway disease (OAD), note that in general, there is a much greater increase in peak airway pressure in the asthma population. In asthma, peak airway pressures may exceed 50 cmH$_2$O to achieve effective ventilation and normalization of PaCO$_2$. However, given the potential detrimental effects of these marked elevations in pressure and the risks of barotrauma or hemodynamic sequellae, strategies of controlled hypoventilation allowing an acceptable increase in PaCO$_2$ but utilizing hyperoxic concentrations of inspired oxygen are often adapted, while the primary therapies directed at reducing the marked increases in Raw are given time to achieve therapeutic effect, thus minimizing ventilator-associated complications (Darioli 1984; Marini 2011). The main goal of mechanical ventilation remains to sustain survivable blood/gas tensions, both PaO$_2$ and PaCO$_2$, with the acceptance of some degree of hypercapnia (termed permissive hypercapnia) within an acceptable range while administering sufficient concentrations of inspired oxygen to maintain adequate system oxygen delivery (Tuxen 1994). In cases of patients with acute asthma and respiratory failure, such a mechanical ventilator strategy might include utilization of controlled mechanical ventilation with high-level sedation at set respiratory rates of approximately 10/minute, reduced tidal volumes in range of 6–8 mL/kg, rapid inspiratory flow rates of 80–100 L/min, and 100 percent FiO_2 to maintain the most important arterial variable—that is, oxygen saturation (Brenner 2009).

In contrast to patients with asthma and ARF, such marked increases in peak airway pressure (Ppeak)—barring acute pneumothorax or major airway mucus plugging—are usually not evident in patients with COPD requiring invasive mechanical ventilation, and thus this controlled hypoventilation strategy is less often needed. In fact, overvigorous ventilation in patients with severe COPD and chronic compensated hyprercarbic respiratory acidosis with compensatory elevations in serum bicarbonate can lead to the development of acute and severe potentially life-threatening acute mechanical ventilation–induced respiratory alkalosis (termed posthypercapnic hyperventilation), which must be avoided because of the potential complications of seizures and cardiac arrhythmias.

In comparison to measurements of respiratory system elastance (Ers) and Raw in healthy subjects, measuring approximately 10 cmH_2O/L and 1.5 $cmH_2O/L/sec$, respectively, physiological measurements of lung mechanics obtained in a cohort of patients with COPD requiring mechanical ventilation demonstrated the following values: Ers (cmH_2O/L) = 23.5 (range 14.6–48.9) and Raw ($cmH_2O/L/Sec$) = 18.0 (range 9.9–31.5) (Leung 1997). In a similar cohort of seven patients with severe COPD requiring mechanical ventilation, inspiratory pulmonary resistance measured 16.1 +/– 1.5 cm $H_2O/L/sec$ (Petrof 1990). In addition, the specific measurement of Raw of the small terminal airways, defined anatomically as distal airways, of less than 2 mm in internal diameter demonstrated similar abnormal lung mechanics: normal small airways' Raw = 0.7 +/– 0.26 $cmH_2O/L/sec$ versus small Raw in patients with COPD = 2.78–4.59 $cmH_2O/L/sec$.

As expected, given the abnormal lung mechanics, in a group of patients with severe COPD requiring mechanical ventilation, marked increases in measured WOB were recorded with values 17.37 +/– 1.92 to 19.84 +/– 2.78

when expressed as J/minute and 1.61 +/– 0.12 to 1.70 +/– 0.15 when expressed as J/L (Petrof 1990). The overall measurement of the total work of breathing (WOB) was partitioned into the elastic component of inspiratory work (Wiel/Ve) and resistive component of inspiratory work (Wires/Ve), and representative values measured 0.89 +/– 0.08 to 0.94 +/– 0.08 J/L and 0.76 +/– 0.12 to 0.70 +/– 0.07 J/l respectively (recalling that normal values for WOBtotal in healthy nondisease individuals = 0.25–0.75 J/L).

However, as a direct result of the physiological abnormality of increased Raw, which is shared by both severe asthma and severe AECOPD requiring invasive mechanical ventilation, one similarity that can occur as a complication of overvigorous mechanical ventilation in association with severe expiratory airflow limitation is the development of auto-PEEP and dynamic hyperinflation. Marked increase in Raw, inhomogeneity of ventilation distribution, and variable time constants within various lung units often contribute to a failure of equalization of alveolar and airway pressures at end expiration, creating what is referred to as auto-PEEP or intrinsic PEEP (meaning not set as part of the ventilator settings/parameters) because of insufficient time and volume for the exhalation of the entirety of the previously inhaled volume of gas. When exhalation terminates before equilibration can be achieved between airway pressure and alveolar pressure and before the respiratory system achieves its fully relaxed position before the next inspiration begins, then the resulting pressure gradient driving end-expiratory flow persists, generating an intrinsic lung-mediated additional positive pressure at end expiration, called auto or intrinsic PEEP [PEEPi] (Marini 2011, Figure 1).

Auto-PEEP is a dynamic process with variable degrees of end-expiratory pressure throughout the myriad of functional diverse and different pulmonary airways given variability in regional time constants, which make the development of auto-PEEP not uniformly distributed throughout the lung (Marini 1989). In settings of severe airflow obstruction, there exists significant inhomogeneity in airway resistance leading to regional differences in time constants and the filling and emptying of lung units, causing variable values of regional volumes and pressures (Leatherman 1996).

The physiological detrimental effects of this intrinsically generated end-expiratory positive pressure are multiple. The creation of hyperinflation and increases in end-expiratory lung volumes (EELV) prior to the onset of the next inspiration can have detrimental hemodynamic consequences by inhibiting venous blood return to the right ventricle. Even more importantly, the increases in EELV can compromise the inspiratory capacity of the lung, as dynamic hyperinflation can increase this volume above the capacity of the relatively stiffer chest wall and thus reduce inspiratory capacity. Auto-PEEP also can compromise the mechanical efficiency of the respiratory muscles by increasing their length-tension relationship to disadvantageous values. Finally, the generation of auto-PEEP can severely hinder weaning since now as spontaneous inspiration begins, the first force or pressures that must be overcome to initiate inspiration and to achieve increases in lung volumes is this added work pressure generated by auto-PEEP. PEEPi once overt, patients must then generate enough pressure to overcome auto-PEEP before inspiration and increases in tidal volume can begin (Georgopoulus 1993). The added stress of mechanical disadvantageous muscle lengths and the necessity for this increased pressure generation can significantly limit the spontaneous ventilatory capacity of already stressed and deconditioned patients in the ICU.

PEEPi can significantly increase the WOB in patients with COPD; for example, a patient who displaces 0.5 L of tidal volume through a 7 cmH_2O pressure gradient will perform an amount of work = 0.35 J/cycle. If nothing else changes, and PEEPi equals 5 cmH_2O, 0.25 J/cycle will be required in addition to maintain that same tidal volume with the accumulated WOB = 0.35 + 0.25 = 0.60 J/cycle, which now represents 40 percent of the entire inspiratory work (Cabello 2006).

As previously discussed, chest wall hyperinflation and hyperexpansion can also significantly increase the overall work of breathing due to the hypocompliance of the chest wall and severely limit the ability for further lung expansion/inflation. During mechanical ventilation, dynamic hyperinflation (DH) is also resultant from insufficient time during expiration for complete exhalation of the delivered tidal volume, causing an increase in the end-expiratory lung volume (EELV) and the generation of auto-PEEP resultant from an increase in alveolar pressure at end-expiration. The key determinant of EELV in ventilated patients are the time constants of the respiratory system (resistance × compliance) and Vt/V̇e ratio imposed by the ventilator settings. To measure the severity of hyperinflation in patients receiving mechanical ventilation, it is necessary to measure the total exhaled volume during a prolonged period of apnea. With this technique, the total amount of gas exhaled during this prolonged apnea represents the volume above FRC at end inspiration (Vei). The volume at end expiration (Vee) is then calculated by subtracting the tidal volume from Vei (Vee = Vei − Vt), and Vee then represents the increase in lung volume caused by dynamic hyperinflation.

The known variables that contribute to DH and auto-PEEP are increased airway resistance, long inspiratory duty times, reduced time for exhalation, and high minute ventilation. Thus therapeutic mechanical ventilation strategies aimed at reducing these factors are efficacious in avoiding or at least minimizing this potential complication. Obviously, for any acute illness, treating the primary pathophysiological process is also first line and foremost in terms of immediate therapy both to assist with ventilator management and also for clinical benefit. Strategies to avoid auto-PEEP and hyperinflation include (a) reduction in respiratory rate to allow greater time for exhalation, (b) reduction in tidal volume to allow less inhaled volume to be appropriately balanced to exhaled volume, and (c) shortening of inspiratory time by increasing inspiratory flow rates to allow greater time for exhalation during each breathing cycle (Brenner 2009). In one study of intubated patients with both asthma and COPD, the largest reductions in end-expiratory lung volumes (Vee/EELV) and thus hyperinflation were demonstrated when expiratory times were increased by reducing RR at constant Vt and inspiratory flow rates (Tuxen 1987, Figure 2). In this study, minute ventilation (V̇e) was the most important determinant of increased volume at end expiration (Vee); but for any given V̇e, dynamic hyperinflation was reduced the most by reductions in RR.

Note that especially in asthma, there exists almost always a component of gas trapping that is anatomically fixed in volume beyond obstructed and occluded airways that will (a) not be able to participate in gas exchange and (b) be a relatively fixed component of Vee until the primary disease process is treated and resolved. The clinical significance of these factors is that for any given set of respiratory variables and parameters, there exists an ideal duty time (Ti/Ttot) to maximize alveolar ventilation (V̇A) for any given RR.

Minute ventilation (V̇e) is a complex function of mechanical ventilator–applied pressure, respiratory rate, compliance, duty time, and regional time constants for both inflation and deflation (Marini 1989). Thus, for any combination of compliance and ventilator preset pressure, the presence of auto-PEEP will limit the tidal volume (Vt) that can be achieved (Marini 1989). Consequently, as RR increases, especially in patients with severe airflow obstruction, the difference between the driving pressure (i.e., preset ventilator pressure minus auto-PEEP) will decrease, eventually reaching a point where Vt will decline and in essence offset any anticipated increase in V̇e achieved or expected by increasing RR or breath frequency (Marini 1989, Figures 4, 6; Amato 2006, Figure 10-4).

References

Amato, M. B. P., and J. J. Marini. 2006. "Pressure-Controlled and Inverse-Ratio Ventilation." In M. J. Tobin, *Principles and Practice of Mechanical Ventilation*. New York: McGraw-Hill, Medical Publishing Division. 251–272.

Begin, P., and A. Grassino. 1991. "Inspiratory Muscle Dysfunction and Chronic Hypercapnia in Chronic Obstructive Pulmonary Disease." *American Review of Respiratory Disease* 143: 905–912.

Brenner, B., T. Corbridge, A. Kazzi. 2009. "Intubation and Mechanical Ventilation of the Asthmatic Patient in Respiratory Failure." *Proceedings of the American Thoracic Society* 6: 371–379.

Brochard, L., J. Mancebo, M. Wysocki, F. Lofasa, G. Conti, A. Rauss, G. Simonneau, et al. 1995. "Noninvasive Ventilation for Acute Exacerbations of Chronic Obstructive Pulmonary Disease." *New England Journal of Medicine* 333: 817–822.

Cabello, B., and J. Mancebo. 2006. "Work of Breathing." *Intensive Care Medicine* 32 (9): 1311–1314.

Celli, B. R., and W. MacNee. 2004. "Standards for the Diagnosis and Treatment of Patients with COPD: A Summary of the ATS/ERS Position Paper." *European Respiratory Journal* 23: 932–946.

Chandra, D., J. A. Stamm, B. Taylor, R. M. Ramos, L. Satterwhite, J. A. Krishan, D. Mannino, et al. 2012. "Outcomes of Noninvasive Ventilation for Acute Exacerbations of Chronic Obstructive Pulmonary Disease in the United States, 1998–2008." *American Journal of Respiratory and Critical Care Medicine* 185 (2): 152–159.

Cohen, L., X. E. J. Tarsi, T. Ramkumar, T. K. Horiuchi, R. Cochran, S. DeMartino, K. B. Schechtman, et al. 2007. "Epithelial Cell Proliferation Contributes to Airway Remodeling in Severe Asthma." *American Journal of Respiratory and Critical Care Medicine* 176: 138–145.

Darioli, R., and C. Perret. 1984. "Mechanical Controlled Hypoventilation in Status Asthmaticus." *American Review of Respiratory Disease* 129: 385–387.

Dhand, R., A. Jubran, and M. J. Tobin 1995. "Bronchodilator Delivery by Metered-Dose Inhaler in Ventilator Supported Patients." *American Journal of Respiratory and Critical Care Medicine* 151: 1827–1833.

Dick, C. R., Z. Liu, C. S. H. Sassoon, R. B. Berry, and C. K. Mahutte. 1997. "O_2-Induced Change in Ventilation and Ventilator Drive in COPD." *American Journal of Respiratory and Critical Care Medicine* 155: 609–614.

Eldridge, F., and C. Gherman. 1968. "Studies of Oxygen Administration in Respiratory Failure." *Annals of Internal Medicine* 68 (3): 569–578.

Fernandez-Perez, E. R., and R. D. Hubmayr. 2006. "Interpretation of Airway Pressure Forms." *Intensive Care Medicine* 32: 658–659.

Ferrer, A., J. Roca, P. D. Wagner, F. A. Lopez, and R. Rodriguez-Roisin. 1993. "Airway Obstruction and Ventilation-Perfusion Relationships in Acute Severe Asthma." *American Review of Respiratory Disease* 147: 579–584.

Gattinonni, L., P. Caironi, M. Cressoni, D. Chiumello, M. Ranieri, M. Quintel, S. Russo, et al. 2006. "Lung Recruitment in Patients with the Acute Respiratory Distress Syndrome." *New England Journal of Medicine* 354: 1775–1786.

Georgopoulos, D., E. Giannouli, and D. Patakas. 1993. "Effects of Extrinsic Positive End-Expiratory Pressure on Mechanically Ventilated Patients with Chronic Obstructive Pulmonary Disease and Dynamic Hyperinflation." *Intensive Care Medicine* 19: 197–203.

Global Initiative for Chronic Obstructive Lung Disease. Updated 2014. www.goldcopd.org.

Hanson, C. W., B. E. Marshall, H. F. Frasch, and P. Marshall. 1996. "Causes of Hypercarbia with Oxygen Therapy in Patients with Chronic Obstructive Pulmonary Disease." *Critical Care Medicine* 24 (1): 23–28.

Jarjour, N. N., S. C. Erzurum, E. R. Bleecker, W. J. Calhoun, M. Castro, S. A. A. Comhair, K. F. Chung, et al. 2012. "Severe Asthma." *American Journal of Respiratory and Critical Care Medicine* 185 (4): 356–362.

Jubran, A., and M. J. Tobin. 1996. "Monitoring during Mechanical Ventilation." *Clinics in Chest Medicine* 17 (3): 453–473.

Kelsen, S. G., and C. J. Criner. 1998. "Pump Failure: The Pathogenesis of Hypercapnic Respiratory Failure in Patients with Lung and Chest Wall Disease." In *Fishman's Pulmonary Disease and Disorders*, edited by A. P. Fishman. New York: McGraw-Hill, Health Professions Division. 2603–2625.

Leatherman, J. W. 1996. "Mechanical Ventilation in Obstructive Lung Disease." *Clinics in Chest Medicine* 17 (3): 577–590.

Leatherman, J. W., C. McArthur, and R. S. Shapiro. 2004. "Effect of Prolongation of Expiratory Time on Dynamic Hyperinflation in Mechanically Ventilated Patients with Severe Asthma." *Critical Care Medicine* 32 (7): 1542–1545.

Leung, P., A. Jubran, and M. J. Tobin. 1997. "Comparison of Assisted Ventilator Modes on Triggering, Patient Effort, and Dyspnea." *American Journal of Respiratory and Critical Care Medicine* 155: 1940–1948.

Loring, S. H., M. Garcia-Jacques, and A. Malhotra. 2009. "Pulmonary Characteristics in COPD and Mechanism of Increased Work of Breathing." *Journal of Applied Physiology* 107 (1): 309–314.

Lotvall, J., C. A. Akdis, L. B. Bacharier, L. Biermer, T. B. Casale, A. Custovic, R. F. Lemaske, et al. 2011. "Asthma Endotypes: A New Approach to Classification of Disease Entities within the Same

Asthma Syndrome." *Journal of Allergy and Clinical Immunology* 127 (2): 355–360.

Marini, J. J. 2011. "Dynamic Hyperinflation and Auto-Positive End-Expiratory Pressure." *American Journal of Respiratory and Critical Care Medicine* 184: 756–762.

Marini, J. J., P. S. Crooke, and J. D. Truwit. 1989. "Determinants and Limits of Pressure-Preset Ventilation: A Mathematical Model of Pressure Control." *Journal of Applied Physiology* 67 (3): 1081–1092.

Marthan, R., Y. Castaing, G. Manier, and H. Guenard. 1985. "Gas Exchange Alterations in Patients with Chronic Obstructive Lung Disease. *Chest* 87 (4): 470–475.

McFadden, E. R. 2003. "Acute Severe Asthma." *American Journal of Respiratory and Critical Care Medicine* 168: 740–759.

McDonough, J.E., R. Yuan, M. Suzuki, N. Seyednejad, W.M. Elliott, P.G. Sanchez, A.C. Wright, et. al. 2011. "Small-airway Obstruction and Emphysema in Chronic Obstructive Pulmonary Disease." *New England Journal of Medicine* 365: 1567-1575.

Moore, W. C., S. C. Erzurum, E. R. Bleecker, B. T. Ameredes, L. Bacharier, M. P. Clark, M. Hew, et al. 2007. "Characterization of the Severe Asthma Phenotype by the National Heart, Lung, and Blood Institute's Severe Asthma Research Program." *Journal of Allergy and Clinical Immunology* 119: 405–413.

O'Donnell, D. E., C. D'Arsigny, M. Fitzpatrick, and K. A. Webb. 2002. "Exercise Hypercapnia in Advanced Chronic Obstructive Pulmonary Disease." *American Journal of Respiratory and Critical Care Medicine* 166: 663–668.

Ordonez, C. L., T. E. Shaughnessy, M. A. Matthay, and J. V. Fahy 2000. "Increased Neutrophil Numbers and IL-8 Levels in Airway Secretions in Acute Severe Asthma." *American Journal of Respiratory and Critical Care Medicine* 161: 1185–1190.

Petrof, B. J., M. Legare, P. Goldberg, J. Milic-Emili, S. and B. Gottfried. 1990. "Continuous Positive Airway Pressure Reduces Work of Breathing and Dyspnea during Weaning from Mechanical Ventilation in Severe Chronic Obstructive Pulmonary Disease." *American Review of Respiratory Disease* 141: 281–289.

Ranieri, V. M., S. Grasso, L. Mascia, S. Martino, T. Fiore, A. Brienza, and R. Giuliani. 1997. "Effects of Proportional Assist Ventilation on Inspiratory Muscle Effort in Patients with Chronic Obstructive Pulmonary Disease and Acute Respiratory Failure." *Anesthesiology* 86 (1): 79–91.

Robinson, T. D., D. B. Freiberg, J. E. Regnis, and I. H. Young. 2000. "The Role of Hypoventilation and Ventilation-Perfusion Redistribution in Oxygen-Induced Hypercapnia during Acute Exacerbations of Chronic Obstructive Pulmonary Disease." *American Journal of Respiratory and Critical Care Medicine* 161: 1524–1529.

Roca, J., R. Rodriguez-Roisin, E. Ballester, J. M. Montserrat, and P. D. Wagner. 1988. "Serial Relationships between Ventilation-Perfusion Inequality and Spirometry in Acute Severe Asthma Requiring Hospitalization." *American Review of Respiratory Disease* 137: 1055–1061.

Rodrigo, G. J., C. Rodrigo, and J. B. Hall. 2004. "Acute Asthma in Adults." *Chest* 125: 1081–1102.

Rodriguez-Roisin, R., E. Ballester, J. Roca, A. Torres, and P. D. Wagner. 1989. "Mechanisms of Hypoxemia in Patients with Status Asthmaticus

Requiring Mechanical Ventilation." *American Review of Respiratory Disease* 139: 732–739.

Rodriguez-Roisin, R., M. Drakulovic, D. A. Rodriguez, J. Roca, J. A. Barbera, and P. D. Wagner. 2009. "Ventilation-Perfusion Imbalance and Chronic Obstructive Pulmonary Disease Staging Severity." *Journal of Applied Physiology* 106: 1902–1908.

Rubinfeld, A. R., P. D. Wagner, J. B. West, and R. C. Matthews 1978. "Gas Exchange during Acute Experimental Canine Asthma." *American Review of Respiratory Disease* 118: 525–535.

Schumaker, G. L., and S. K. Epstein. 2004. "Managing Acute Respiratory Failure during Exacerbation of Chronic Obstructive Pulmonary Disease." *Respiratory Care* 49 (7): 766–782.

Singer, B. D., and T. C. Corbridge. 2009. "Basic Invasive Mechanical Ventilation." *Southern Medical Journal* 102 (12): 1238–1245.

Soler-Cataluna, J. J., M. A. Martinez-Garcia, P. Roman Sanchez, E. Salcedo, M. Navarro, and R. Ochando. 2005. "Severe Acute Exacerbations and Mortality in Patients with Chronic Obstructive Pulmonary Disease." *Thorax* 60: 925–931.

Sur, S., T. B. Crotty, G. M. Kephart, B. A. Hyma, T. V. Colby, C. E. Reed, L. W. Hunt, and G. J. Gleich. 1993. "Sudden Onset Fatal Asthma." *American Review of Respiratory Disease* 148: 713–719.

Tobin, M. J. 1988. "Respiratory Monitoring in the Intensive Care Unit." *American Review of Respiratory Disease* 138: 1625–1642.

———. 1990. "Respiratory Monitoring." *JAMA* 264 (2): 244–251.

Tuxen, D. V. 1994. "Permissive Hypercapnic Ventilation." *American Journal of Respiratory and Critical Care Medicine* 150: 870–874.

Tuxen, D. V., and S. Lane. 1987. "The Effects of Ventilatory Pattern on Hyperinflation, Airway Pressures, and Circulation in Mechanical Ventilation of Patients with Severe Air-Flow Obstruction." *American Review of Respiratory Disease* 136: 872–879.

Wagner, P. D., and R. Rodriguez-Roisin. 1991. "Clinical Advances in Pulmonary Gas Exchange." *American Review of Respiratory Disease* 143: 883–888.

Wagner, P. D., D. R. Dantzker, R. Dueck, J. L. Clausen, and J. B. West. 1977. "Ventilation-Perfusion Inequality in Chronic Obstructive Pulmonary Disease." *Journal of Clinical Investigation* 59: 203–216.

Wagner, P. D., D. R. Dantzker, V. E. Iacovoni, W. C. Tomlin, and J. B. West. 1978. "Ventilation-Perfusion Inequality in Asymptomatic Asthma." *American Review of Respiratory Disease* 118: 511–525.

Wagner, P. D., G. Hedenstierna, and G. Bylin. 1987. "Ventilation-Perfusion Inequality in Chronic Asthma." *American Review of Respiratory Disease* 136: 605–612.

Wahidi, M. M., and M. Kraft. 2012. "Bronchial Thermoplasty for Severe Asthma." *American Journal of Respiratory and Critical Care Medicine* 185 (7): 709–714.

Ward, M. E., et al. 1994. "Respiratory Mechanics." In *Textbook of Respiratory Medicine*, edited by J. F. Murray and J. A. Nadel. Philadelphia: W. B. Saunders Company. 90–138.

West, J. B., and P. D. Wagner. 1991. "Ventilation Perfusion Relationships." In *The Lung Scientific Foundations*, edited by R. G. Crystal and J. B. West. New York: Raven Press. 1289–1306.

CHAPTER 15

Acute Respiratory Distress Syndrome

• • •

ARDS IS A CLINICAL SYNDROME of variable causation defined by a combination of clinical, laboratory, and radiographic variables/parameters that include (a) acute onset, (b) P/F ratio (PaO_2 [mmHg]/FiO2 [decimal]) less than 300 mmHg, (c) bilateral infiltrates on standard chest radiograph, and (d) pulmonary capillary wedge pressure (PCWP) or left atrial pressure (LAP) less than 18 mmHg or no clinical evidence of left atrial hypertension (Bernard 1994; ARDS 2011). Perhaps no other disease has generated more intense critical-care scrutiny, investigation, and controversy than ARDS. However, this intensive investigation has generated enormous amounts of clinical information, which can literally be used to track the various eras of critical-care medicine, from the first delineation of this syndrome in 1967 through the Vietnam War (often referred to as Da Nang lung), when it became widely publicized, to the days of "best" positive end-expiratory pressure (PEEP) to "super" PEEP and oxygen toxicity, into the decade of Swan Ganz glory and emphasis upon O_2 delivery and not simply O_2 content, and then into the "lung protection" mechanical ventilation strategy, and finally into the "baby lung" or "sponge lung" scenario, not to mention the innumerable failed pharmacological interventional clinical trials.

ARDS represents a stereotypic, programmed lung-injury response to a wide variety of injurious agents. In addition, it must be noted that ARDS is a dynamic, ongoing disease process with changing day-to-day pathology and pathophysiology and the necessity for near daily and often hourly clinical adjustments including mechanical ventilation settings. Each of these distinct clinical and pathological stages represents unique pathological/anatomical descriptions and resultant unique physiological abnormalities (Matamis 1984). The early injury phases of ARDS are characterized by extensive capillary endothelial cell destruction and total dysfunction of capillary permeability generating hemorrhagic areas of alveolar-capillary wall lung destruction with hemorrhage, predominate neutrophilic inflammatory infiltration, and necrotic debris in the airways, often referred to as hyaline membranes. In contrast to cardiogenic hydrostatic pulmonary edema, where lymphatic and alveolar fluid composition reflects transudative characteristics, in permeability edema, ARDS, due to the total disruption of capillary filtering and restricting capacity alveolar fluid, tends to reflect exudative characteristics with high concentrations of acute inflammatory cells and profibrotic, proinflammatory, procoagulant factors. The next pathological stage represents the lungs' response to injury and efforts to initiate repair with the development of intense mononuclear cell organization. Finally dense fibrosis leading to totally irreversible lung destruction and total effacement of normal-appearing tissue can develop in up to 10 percent of patients with ARDS. The various signals or components that trigger one phase to the next or the exact time frame from one phase to the next are undefined, but these transitions can either not occur at all, allowing lung recovery to virtually full functionality, or rapidly progress to irreversible and fatal lung fibrosis.

The hallmark pathophysiological characteristics of ARDS are hypocompliant stiff lungs and refractory oxygenation. Although initially believed to be a homogenous disease, it is now very evident and critical to the understanding of the abnormal physiology and subsequent clinical and ventilatory management of ARDS that the disease acute lung injury (ALI)/ARDS is in reality a very inhomogeneous disease with nonhomogenous distributions of pulmonary aeration/ventilation very influenced by gravitational forces and body habitus with (a) areas of relatively normal (noninjured) lung (referred to as the functional "baby" lung), (b) areas of intermediate but still "salvageable" lung with gas-exchanging alveoli, and (c) areas of degassed totally atelectatic collapsed lung units incapable of gas exchange (Slutsky 2005). The importance of gravitational forces and body habitus in contributing to dysfunctional lung units is most evident by the intervention of prone positioning, which, in virtually all patients, achieves improvements in gas exchange and oxygenation status—although no universal beneficial effects upon mortality have been evident, again emphasizing the total body consequences of the disease processes that cause ARDS and the only approximate 5–10 percent lung or respiratory-related mortality for a disease that can carry up to 40–50 percent total overall mortality.

Analysis of computerized tomography (CT) images from intubated patients with ARDS receiving mechanical ventilation have revealed a nonhomogenous distribution of lung patterns in patients with ARDS: (a) hyperinflated, (b) normally aerated, (c) poorly aerated, and (d) nonaerated (Paolo 2007). Normally aerated lungs are relatively small, but when they receive the largest part of tidal volume via mechanical ventilation, they may be exposed to excessive alveolar wall tension and stress because of overdistention and hyperinflation (Grasso 2007; Putensen 2009). Atelectactic lung regions are prone to cyclic recruitment and derecruitment leading to shear stress in adjacent aerated and nonaerated alveoli and the subsequent release of inflammatory mediators that can precipitate multiorgan failure (MOF) or directly cause ventilator-induced lung injury (Putensen 2009). As an aid in understanding, I tend to refer to these different functional lung components as analogous to the same concept in relation to an acute cerebral stroke with the central infarcted/necrotic area, the surrounding potentially salvageable penumbra, and the outer border of normal functional neuronal tissues.

Abnormal Gas Exchange in ARDS

Refractory hypoxemia (defined as P/F < 300) is a requirement for the delineation of the clinical syndrome ARDS. Again utilizing the MIGET technique, marked elevations in true shunt fraction (defined as V/Q < 0.005) have been observed in virtually all patients with values ranging from 18 to 68 percent of total cardiac output. In addition, in relation to hypoxemia, ARDS represents one of the few critical-care diseases whereby pure shunt physiology (37 +/− 14% and 45 +/− 17%) often dominates as the predominate mechanism (Caironi 2010). The presence of these large intrapulmonary shunts easily explains the profound hypoxemia of ARDS not responsive to even high concentrations of inspired oxygen. Experimental animal models of validated ARDS injury demonstrated similar results, with 16.5 percent of total pulmonary blood flow attributed to true shunt V/Q values (Wagner 1975; West 1991, Figure 12).

In addition, most patients demonstrate a significant volume of lung units with abnormally low V/Q ratios (defined as 0.005 < V/Q < 0.1). On average, the presence of shunt plus low V/Q shuntlike units accounted for an average of 48 percent of total blood flow and easily explains the severe degrees of hypoxemia. In addition, the close agreement between measured PaO_2 and predicted arterial PaO_2 using MIGET in select groups of ARDS patients strongly argues against significant diffusion impairment as cause of hypoxemia in ARDS (Dantzker 1979; Melot 1994). In summary, the V/Q units in patients with ARDS demonstrate two distinct ranges: (a) 52 percent of cardiac output perfused by lung units with relatively normal preserved V/Q ratios and (b) 48 percent of CO to previously noted units with low V/Q rations, representing either true shunt or very low V/Q ratios (increased venous admixture $\dot{Q}s/\dot{Q}t$).

Often lost in the emphasis upon oxygenation is the additional fact that in almost all ARDS patients, there also exists a marked increase in deadspace ventilation, with studies demonstrating dead space to tidal volume fractions (Vd/Vt) equaling 42+/− 9 percent (Gattinoni 2006); 37 +/− 14 percent, and 45 +/− 17 percent (Caironi 2010). This same study showed this calculation has validity as a marker of increased mortality as shown in Table 15.1 (Gattinoni 2006). However, compensatory increases in minute ventilation ($\dot{V}e$), either spontaneous or mechanical ventilator–induced, are usually more than effective in overcoming these still significant increases in Vd/Vt so as to maintain normal levels of $PaCO_2$, unless patients progress to the development of severe, irreversible, diffuse lung fibrosis. Again of note, in patients with ARDS, true shunt is almost always observed (Dantzker 1979).

Table 15.1: Pulmonary Physiological Measurements in Survivors and Nonsurvivors of Acute Respiratory Distress Syndrome (ARDS) (Gattinoni 2006)

	Vd/Vt	Cresp mL/cmH₂O	Qs/Qt (shunt fraction)
ARDS Survivors	53 +/− 12%	51 +/− 19	34 +/− 12%
ARDS Nonsurvivors	63 +/− 13%	38+/− 15	45 +/− 17%

The mortality prognostic/predictive value of serial measurements of Vd/Vt in multiple groups of critically ill patients requiring invasive mechanical ventilation, including ARDS, was again recently substantiated (Frankenfield 2010; Vender 2014). This publication again supported the apparent identified threshold values for Vd/Vt that reliably predicted survival (Vd/Vt < 50 percent) compared to nonsurvival (Vd/Vt > 65 percent).

Abnormal Respiratory Mechanics in ARDS

The analysis of pressure-volume (P-V) curves in either human patients with ARDS or valid experimental animal models of acute lung injury (ALI) are remarkably similar and again somewhat reflective of the P-V relationship of the normal, nondiseased, healthy lung. Pulmonary physiological measurements from mechanical ventilation in patients with ARDS have demonstrated the existence of an early inspiratory phase of initially poorly distensible lung tissue that requires a relatively large head of driving pressure to effect even a small amount of increase in tidal volume from end expiration—termed the flat lower portion of the ARDS P-V loop. There then follows a relatively steep phase of inflation, which encompasses the vast majority of this sigmoidal or S-shaped P-V curve. The transition between this initial flat portion of the P-V curve and the beginning of the steep hypercompliant portion of the P-V curve is referred to as the lower inflection point (LIP). At end inspiration and near full tidal volume, the P-V curve again becomes relatively flat in its upper portion of the curve, with this flat upper portion representing areas of alveoli that are being overdistended and stretched beyond their usual expected volumes (Slutsky 2005, Figure 8). The transition point in the P-V curve between these two latter volume transitions is referred to as the upper inflection point (UIP). In summary, this sigmoid shape of inflation P-V curve in patients with ARDs tends to create two inflection points: relatively hypocompliant lower and upper portions and finally the middle portion of "best" compliance (Matamis 1984, Figure 3; Hickling 2002; Slutsky 2005). However in patients progressing to severe lung fibrosis as a sequellae of ARDS, the hypercompliant phase of the P-V curve tends to be eliminated with resultant relatively flat and linear characteristics (Matamis 1984).

Various physiological calculations can be made referencing the pressure measurements recorded from the manometers or graphic displays of the mechanical ventilator. The static compliance of the respiratory system (Cst, resp) can be calculated at zero flow by dividing tidal volume of a mechanically delivered breath/inspiration by the difference of the plateau pressure (obtained following a 0.5-second inspiratory pause) and end-expiratory pressure often measured as total PEEP; that is, Cst, resp = Vt/(Pplateau − PEEP). Because PEEP is a component of the absolute value of Pplateau, as PEEP increases, Pplateau increases; thus PEEP should be subtracted from Pplateau in the measurement of the total respiratory systems compliance but included in measurements of plateau pressure (Pplat) (Tobin 1988, Figure 6; Tobin 1990; Fernandez-Perez 2006, Figure 1; Singer 2009, Figure 8; Hess 2014, Figure 1).

Using these techniques, in cohorts of patients with ARDS respiratory system compliance (mL/cmH_2O) was measured 46 +/− 16 and 41 +/− 24 (Caironi 2009). Other studies using the same formula for respiratory-systems compliance (mL/cmH_2O) have demonstrated similar abnormally low values in ARDS patients compared to standard control patient populations (i.e., surgical controls 56 +/− 16, medical controls 45 +/− 11, and ARDs patients 42 +/− 14; this latter value is influenced by the standard-of-care accepted techniques of limiting tidal volume to 6 mL/kg or less and Pplateau < 30 cmH$_2$O) [Table 15.2] (Chiumello 2008).

However, what is most marked in this same study is the significant reductions in FRC (functional residual capacity) in the ARDS patients compared to the same control populations (i.e., surgical controls = 1715 +/− 734 mL; medical control = 1166+/−392 mL; and ARDS patients = 1013 +/− 593 mL) (Chiumello 2008). Although not frequently discussed, the lung physiological measurement of FRC may very well be the most important measurement/parameter in the care of critically ill patients, as FRC represents the sump, or reservoir, of O$_2$ stores to continuously provide a gradient for the uptake of O$_2$ from the alveolar gas into the alveolar capillary and the red blood cell (RBC). These reductions in FRC were linearly related to and resultant from decreases in lung compliance (Katz 1981). Most critical-care physicians are well aware of the phenomenon of the "gasless" lung, whereby in the absence of an alveolar reserve of O$_2$ to be taken up by the RBCs in the alveolar capillaries or in presence of severely reduced levels of FRC, arterial oxygen levels can fall precipitously to values approaching mixed venous almost instantaneously (Fan 2008).

Table 15.2: Pulmonary Physiological Measurements in Patients with Acute Respiratory Distress Syndrome (ARDS) (Chiumello 2008)

	Control (surgical)	Control (medical)	ALI	ARDS
Respiratory system Compliance (mL/cmH$_2$O)	56 +/− 16	45 +/− 11	47 +/− 18	42 +/− 14
FRC (mL)	1715 +/− 734	1166 +/− 392	1088 +/− 391	1013 +/− 593

Finally, Fan (2008) measured total respiratory system compliance at 34 +/− 4.5 mL/cmH$_2$O, and Gattinoni (2006) measured respiratory system compliance at 44 +/− 17 mL/cmH$_2$O in ARDS patients. These marked reductions in total respiratory-systems compliance (Crs, total) result primarily from reductions in lung compliance (Clung) with preserved measurements near normal values for chest-wall compliance (Ccw): Crs, total = 30 mL/cm-H_2O (range 26–35); Ccw = 125 mL/cmH_2O (range 105–146); and Clung = 43 mL/cmH_2O (range 36–50) (Kallet 2007).

Ventilator strategies have evolved based upon these various physiological principles, and the recognition that overdistention of relatively normal compliant lung can lead to lung injury/trauma and possible extra-alveolar air. These ventilator strategies are also based on the fact that sheer stresses from the recurrent opening and closing of vulnerable airspaces can cause direct lung injury, and the elaboration of chemokines/cytokines can be extremely harmful proinflammatory agents/mediators that lead not only to local further escalation of lung injury but also to inflammatory mediated distal multiorgan failure (MOF) (ARDSNet 2000). Others have argued that no absolute value of tidal volume (Vt) per se but rather maintaining the Pplateau less than 30 cmH_2O is the key to avoiding barotrauma (development of extra-alveolar air), volutrauma (often termed ventilator-induced lung injury), or biotrauma (lung generated production of inflammatory mediators) in patients with ARDS.

Recent studies have attempted to refine the relationship between tidal volume (Vt), positive end-expiratory pressure (PEEP), and implementation of the lung protection ventilation strategy upon multiple clinical outcomes in critically ill and post-operative patients requiring invasive mechanical ventilation. Two publications analyzing previously reported clinical trials data in patients with ARDS and post-operative patients have shown a relationship between higher levels of a calculated derived value termed "driving pressure" and worse clinical outcomes (Amato 2015; Neto 2016). By definition, driving pressure equals Vt/Crs which in effect is calculated as the difference between the ventilator induced plateau pressure (Pplat) and the level of PEEP (Pplat — PEEP). Specifically, analyses of this retrospective data seemed to indicate that there were thresholds for driving pressure above which there was a relationship between higher driving pressures and mortality in ARDS patients and a composite term of pulmonary complications in post-operative patients. These speculations still require formal confirmation and validation in well-designed prospective and randomized clinical trials but merit comment.

Thus, strategies to prevent derecruitment (i.e., PEEP) and to avoid overdistention (i.e., Pplat < 30 cmH$_2$O) have now become standards of ventilatory management of the ARDS patient with proven benefits in relation to improved survival (ARDSnet 2000). However, at all times, it must be acknowledged that there are universally severely damaged areas of the lung, mostly in posterior and gravity-dependent portions of the ARDS patient, which for the immediate period are lost and totally incapable of effective gas exchange and totally incapable of undergoing recruitment and expansion or reopening, despite even excessive levels of inspiratory pressures (often exceeding 50 cmH$_2$O). These totally dysfunctional alveolar units result not only for alveolar flooding with exudative inflammatory debris but also the inability of damaged type II pneumocytes to generate surfactant critically necessary for alveolar stability.

Recruitment refers to the dynamic process of reopening unstable airless alveoli through an intentional transient increase in transpulmonary pressure with putative benefits by preventing repetitive opening and closing of unstable lung units. However, the degree or magnitude of recruitable lung is highly variable from ARDS patient to patient, with one study showing 17 percent of patients with recruitable lung volumes between 0 and 25 percent, 50 percent of patients with recruitable lung volumes between 25 and 50 percent, 30 percent with recruitable lung volumes between 50 and 75 percent, and 3 percent with values above 75 percent (Gattinoni 2006).

This same study reported important survival prognostic differences for physiological variables recorded from parameters obtained during invasive mechanical ventilation. In fact, the maintenance of *stable* Pplateau in the first forty-eight hours of ARDS after accounting for tidal volume is a respiratory-system-specific value that carries strong prognostic significance (Checkley 2008): the adjusted odds ratio of death was 1.17 times greater when preenrollment Pplateau increased from 15 to 20 cmH$_2$O, 1.37 times greater when preenrollment Pplateau increased from 20 to 30 cmH$_2$O, and 1.87 greater when preenrollment Plat increased from 30 to 50 cmH$_2$O (Checkley 2008).

As a result of these severe derangements in both gas exchange and lung mechanics, the spontaneous breathing pattern for patients with ARDS is characterized by tachypnea, reduced vital volume (Vt), and increased RR, often progressing to the requirement for invasive mechanical ventilator support. As previously noted, this progression to respiratory failure is the direct consequence of marked increases in WOB that are unable to be sustained by the respiratory muscles (Kallet 2007). Values for these various physiological parameters measured in critically ill patients are recorded as follows:

WOB (total) = 1.60 J/L (1.34–1.85)
WOB (elastic) = 0.92 J/L (0.76–1.08)
WOB (resistive) = 0.68 J/L (0.56–0.80)
WOB elastic/total = 57% (54–61)
WOB resistive/total = 43% (39–46)

REFERENCES

Amato, M.B.P., M.O. Meade, A.S. Slutsky, L. Brochard, E.L.V. Costa, D.A. Schoenfeld, T.E. Stewart, et. al. 2015. "Driving Pressure and Survival in the Acute Respiratory Distress Syndrome." *New England Journal of Medicine* 372: 747-755.

ARDS Definition Task Force. 2012. "Acute Respiratory Distress Syndrome: The Berlin Definition." *Journal of the American Medical Association* 307: 2526–2533.

Bernard, G. R., A. Artigas, K. L. Brigham, J. Carlet, K. Falke, L. Hudson, and M. Lamy. 1994. "The American-European Consensus Conference on ARDS." *American Journal of Respiratory and Critical Care Medicine* 149: 818–824.

Caironi, P., M. Cressoni, D. Chiumello, M. Ranieri, M. Quintel, S.G. Russo, R. Cornejo, et al. 2010. "Lung Opening and Closing during Ventilation of Acute Respiratory Distress Syndrome." *American Journal of Respiratory and Critical Care Medicine* 181: 578–586.

Checkley, W., R. Brower, A. Korpak, B. Taylor Thompson. 2008. "Effects of a Clinical Trial on Mechanical Ventilation Practices in Patients with Acute Lung Injury." *American Journal of Respiratory and Critical Care Medicine* 177: 1215–1222.

Chiumello, D., E. Carlesso, P. Cadringher, P. Caironi, F. Valenza, F. Polli, F. Tallarini, et al. 2008. "Lung Stress and Strain during Mechanical Ventilation for Acute Respiratory Distress Syndrome." *American Journal of Respiratory and Critical Care Medicine* 178: 346–355.

Dantzker, D. R., C. J. Brook, P. Dehart, J. P. Lynch, and J. G. Weg. 1979. "Ventilation-Perfusion Distributions in Adult Respiratory Distress Syndrome." *American Review of Respiratory Disease* 120: 1039–1052.

Fan, E., M. E. Wilcox, R. G. Brower, T. E. Stewart, S. Mehta, S. E. Lapinsky, M. O. Meade, and N. D. Ferguson. 2008. "Recruitment Maneuvers for Acute Lung Injury." *American Journal of Respiratory and Critical Care Medicine* 178: 1156–1163.

Fernandez-Perez, E. R., and R. D. Hubmayr. 2006. "Interpretation of Airway Pressure Waveforms." *Intensive Care Medicine* 32: 658–659.

Frankenfield, D. C., S. Alam, E. Bekteshi, and R. L. Vender. 2010 "Predicting Dead Space Ventilation in Critically Ill Patients Using Clinically Available Data." *Critical Care Medicine* 38: 288–291.

Gattinoni, L., P. Caironi, M. Cressoni, D. Chiumello, M. Ranieri, M. Quintel, S. Russo, et al. 2006. "Lung Recruitment in Patients with the Acute Respiratory Distress Syndrome." *New England Journal of Medicine* 354: 1775–1786.

Gattinoni, L., A. Protti, P. Caironi, and E. Carlesso. 2010. "Ventilator-Induced Lung Injury: The Anatomic and Physiological Framework." *Critical Care Medicine* 38 (10): S539–S548.

Grasso, S., T. Stripoli, M. De Michele, F. Bruno, M. Moschetta, G. Angelelli, I. Munno, et al. 2007. "ARDSnet Ventilator Protocol and Alveolar Hyperinflation." *American Journal of Respiratory and Critical Care Medicine* 176: 761–767.

Hess, D. R. 2014. "Respiratory Mechanics in Mechanically Ventilated Patients." *Respiratory Care* 59 (11): 1773–1794.

Hickling, K. G. 2002. "Reinterpreting the Pressure-Volume Curve in Patients with Acute Respiratory Distress Syndrome." *Current Opinions in Critical Care* 8: 32–38.

Kallet, R. H., J. C. Hemphill, R. A. Dicker, J. A. Alonso, A. R. Campbell, R. C. Mackersie, and J. A. Katz. 2007. "The Spontaneous Breathing Pattern and Work of Breathing of Patients with Acute Respiratory Distress Syndrome and Acute Lung Injury." *Respiratory Care* 52: 989–995.

Katz, J. A., S. E. Zinn, G. M. Ozanne, and H. B. Fairley. 1981. "Pulmonary, Chest Wall, and Lung-Thorax Elastances in Acute Respiratory Failure." *Chest* 80 (3): 304–311.

Matamis, D., F. Lemaire, A. Harf, C. Brun-Buisson, J. C. Ansquer, and G. Atlan. 1984. "Total Respiratory Pressure-Volume Curves in the Adult Respiratory Distress Syndrome." *Chest* 86 (1): 58–66.

Melot, C. 1994. "Ventilation Perfusion Relationships in Acute Respiratory Failure. *Thorax* 49: 1251–1258.

Neto, A.S., S. N. T. Hemmes, C.S.V. Barbas, M. Beiderlinden, A.F. Fernandez-Bustamante, E. Futier, O. Gajic, et. al. 2016. "Association between Driving Pressure and Development of Postoperative Pulmonary Complications in Patients Undergoing Mechanical Ventilation for General Anesthesia: A Meta-analysis of Individual Patient Data." *Lancet Respiratory Medicine* 4: 272-280.

Terragni, P. P., G. Rosboch, A. Tealdi, E. Corno, E. Menaldo, O. Davini, G. Gandini, et al. 2007. "Tidal Hyperinflation during Low Tidal Volume Ventilation in Acute Respiratory Distress Syndrome." *American Journal of Respiratory and Critical Care Med* 175: 160–166.

Putensen, C., N. Theuerkauf, J. Zinserling, H. Wrigge, and P. Pelosi. 2009. "Meta-Analysis: Ventilation Strategies and Outcomes of the Acute Respiratory Distress Syndrome and Acute Lung Injury." *Annals of Internal Medicine* 151: 566–576.

Singer, B. D., and T. C. Corbridge. 2009. "Basic Invasive Mechanical Ventilation." *Southern Medical Journal* 102 (12): 1238–1245.

Slutsky, A. 2005. "Ventilator-Induced Lung Injury: From Barotrauma to Biotrauma." *Respiratory Care* 50 (5): 646–659.

The Acute Respiratory Distress Syndrome Network. 2000. "Ventilation with Lower Tidal Volumes as Compared with Traditional Tidal Volumes for Acute Lung Injury and the Acute Respiratory Distress Syndrome." *New England Journal of Medicine* 342: 1301–1308.

Tobin, M. J. 1988. "Respiratory Monitoring in the Intensive Care Unit." *American Review of Respiratory Disease* 138: 1625–1642.

Tobin, M. J. 1990. "Respiratory Monitoring." *Journal of the American Medical Association* 264 (2): 244–251.

Vender, R. L., M. F. Betancourt, E. B. Lehman, C. Harrell, D. Galvan, and D. C. Frankenfield. 2014. "Prediction Equation to Estimate Dead Space to Tidal Volume Fraction Correlates with Mortality in Critically Ill Patients." *Journal of Critical Care* 29 (2): e1–317e3.

Wagner, P. D., R. B. Laravuso, E. Goldzimmer, P. F. Nauman, and J. B. West. 1975. "Distributions of Ventilation-Perfusion Ratios in Dogs with Normal and Abnormal Lungs." *Journal of Applied Physiology* 38 (6): 1099–1109.

West, J. B., and P. D. Wagner. 1991. "Ventilation Perfusion Relationships." In *The Lung Scientific Foundations*, edited by R. G. Crystal and J. B. West. New York: Raven Press. 1289–1306.

CHAPTER 16

Severe Community-Acquired Pneumonia

• • •

COMMUNITY-ACQUIRED PNEUMONIA (CAP) IS THE most common cause of death associated with infectious disease in the United States (Salluh 2008). More than one million patients with CAP will require hospitalization, and approximately 10–40 percent will require ICU care (Ewig 1998; Restrepo 2010). Although severe CAP (SCAP) is frequently quoted as a specific disease entity in the medical literature, there remains no universally accepted definition of SCAP. Some studies define SCAP as patients requiring ICU care including mechanical ventilation. Other definitions of SCAP rely upon clinical or laboratory parameters to define SCAP, such as requirement for invasive mechanical ventilation, vasopressor hemodynamic support, shock, or various combinations of potentially predictive factors of poor clinical outcomes such as systolic blood pressure, arterial pH, respiratory rate, blood urea nitrogen (BUN), PaO_2, PaO_2/FiO_2, chest x-ray (CXR), age, or altered mental status (delirium, confusion, coma) (Angus 2002; Espana 2006). Regardless of definition, published mortality for patients with diagnosis of severe CAP remains high even with current practice guidelines and established levels of care: 17 percent (Salluh 2008), 24 percent (Rello 2003), 24 percent (Moine 1994), 26 percent (Restrepo 2010), 30 percent (Confalonieri 2005), and 29 percent (Ruiz 1999).

Abnormal Gas Exchange in Acute Bacterial Pneumonia

Hypoxemia is a near-universal finding in cases of acute infectious bacterial pneumonia with mechanistic similarities to previously mentioned disease states, including the importance of staging or timing of acute lung injury and predominate mechanism of hypoxemia resultant from areas of either true shunt (V/Q < 0.005) or, more commonly, increased venous admixture ($Q\dot{}s/Q\dot{}t$) in association with low V/Q relationships (V/Q between 0.005 and 0.1) (Gea 1991, Figure 1). In general, during the early pretreatment acute inflammatory stage, there occurs a shift from lung units with normal V/Q ratios to lung units of low V/Q hypothesized to result from both (a) paralysis of the acute hypoxic vasoconstrictor response so as to maintain perfusion (Q) to the diseased lung segment, often excessive overperfusion given acute inflammation; and (b) reductions in ventilation (V) related to alveolar and airway occlusive infectious debris (Graham 1990; Ferrer 1997). These areas of shunt-directed low V/Q units are accompanied by 10 percent or more of the cardiac output, in some cases as high as 20 percent (Lampron 1985). With recovery there was, as expected, a shift back to lung units with better preserved V/Q relationships and associated improved oxygenation (Wagner 1975). In summary, in cases of SCAP, abnormal gas-exchange physiology was typically associated with a pattern of (a) bimodal V/Q ratio distributions with (1) distinct population of low V/Q units and (2) distinct population with normal V/Q units; and (b) absent to no shunt; and (c) absent to no diffusion impairment (Hanly 1987; Melot 1994).

References

Angus, D. C., T. J. Marrie, D. S. Obrosky, G. Clermont, T. T. Dremsizov, C. Coley, M. J. Fine, D. E. Singer, and W. N. Kapoor. 2002. "Severe Community Acquired Pneumonia." *American Journal of Respiratory and Critical Care Medicine* 166: 717–723.

Confalonieri, M., R. Urbino, A. Potena, M. Piattella, P. Parigi, G. Puccio, R. Della Porta, et al. 1999. "Acute Respiratory Failure in Patients with Severe Community Acquired Pneumonia." *American Journal of Respiratory and Critical Care Medicine* 160: 1585–1591.

Espana, P. P., A. Capelastegui, I. Gorodo, C. Esteban, M. Oribe, M. Ortega, A. Bilbao, and J. M. Quintana. 2006. "Development and Validation of a Clinical Prediction Rule for Severe Community Acquired Pneumonia." *American Journal of Respiratory and Critical Care Medicine* 174: 1249–1256.

Ewig, S., M. Ruiz, J. M. A. Marcos, J. A. Martinez, F. Arancibia, M. S. Niederman, and A. Torres. 1998. "Severe Community Acquired Pneumonia." *American Journal of Respiratory and Critical Care Medicine* 158: 1102–1108.

Ferrer, M., A. Torres, R. Baer, C. Hernandez, J. Roca, and R. Rodriguez-Roisin. 1997. "Effect of Acetylsalicylic Acid on Pulmonary Gas Exchange in Patients with Severe Pneumonia: A Pilot Study." *Chest* 111: 1094–1100.

Gea, J., J. Roca, A. Torres, A. G. N. Agusti, P. D. Wagner, and R. Rodriguez-Roisin. 1991. "Mechanisms of Abnormal Gas Exchange in Patients with Pneumonia." *Anesthesiology* 75: 782–789.

Graham, L. M., A. Vasil, M. L. Vasil, N. F. Voelkel, and K. R. Stenmark. 1990. "Decreased Pulmonary Vaso-Reactivity in an Animal Model of Chronic Pseudomonas Pneumonia." *American Review of Respiratory Disease* 142: 221–229.

Hanly, P., and R. B. Light. 1987. "Lung Mechanics, Gas Exchange, Pulmonary Perfusion, and Hemodynamics in a Canine Model of Acute Pseudomonas Pneumonia." *Lung* 165: 305–322.

Lampron, N., F. Lemaire, B. Teisseire, A. Harf, M. Paolt, D. Matamis, and A. M. Lorino. 1985. "Mechanical Ventilation with 100% Oxygen Does Not Increase Intrapulmonary Shunt in Patients with Severe Bacterial Pneumonia." *American Review of Respiratory Disease* 131: 409–413.

Melot, C. 1994. "Ventilation Perfusion Relationships in Acute Respiratory Failure." *Thorax* 49: 1251–1258.

Moine, P., J-B. Vercken, S. Chevret, C. Chastang, and P. Gajdos. 1994. "Severe Community Acquired Pneumonia, Etiology, Epidemiology, and Prognosis Factors." *Chest* 105: 1487–1495.

Rello, J., M. Bodi, D. Mariscal, M. Navarro, E. Diaz, M. Gallego, and J. Valles. 2003. "Microbiology Testing and Outcome of Patients with Severe Community Acquired Pneumonia." *Chest* 123: 174–180.

Restrepo, M. I., E. M. Mortensen, J. Rello, J. Brody, and A. Anzueto. 2010. "Late Admission to the ICU in Patients with Community Acquired Pneumonia Is Associated with Higher Mortality." *Chest* 137: 552–557.

Ruiz, M., S. Ewig, A. Torres, F. Arancibia, F. Marco, J. Mensa, M. Sanchez, J. A. Martinez. 1999. "Severe Community Acquired Pneumonia." *American Journal of Respiratory and Critical Care Medicine* 160: 923–929.

Salluh, J. I. F., F. A. Bozza, M. Soares, J. C. R. Verdeal, H. C. Castro-Faria-Neto, J. R. Lapa e Silva, and P. T. Bozza. 2008. "Adrenal Response in Severe Community Acquired Pneumonia." *Chest* 134: 947–954.

Wagner, P. D., R. B. Laravuso, E. Goldzimmer, P. F. Naumann, and J. B. West. 1975. "Distributions on Ventilation-Perfusion Ratios in Dogs with Normal and Abnormal Lungs." *Journal of Applied Physiology* 38 (6): 1099–1109.

CHAPTER 17
Blunt Chest Trauma

• • •

Pulmonary Contusion

PULMONARY OR LUNG CONTUSION IS a frequent complication of blunt chest trauma resultant from numerous types and mechanisms of chest injury such as blunt force impact or distant blast injuries. One study quoted a 17 percent incidence of pulmonary contusion in patients with multiple trauma (Cohn 1997). Most of the time, the lung abnormality is secondary in severity in relation to more severe other organ injury/trauma such as head injury, aortic dissection, or even flail chest (Johnson 1986). However, in its severe form, and dependent upon extent of overall profusion and distribution of lung injury, lung contusion remains a risk factor and cause of acute respiratory distress syndrome (ARDS) with associated relatively high respiratory and nonrespiratory mortality (Cohn 1997; Pepe 1982; Hans-Christoph 2000; Miller 2001; Leone 2003; Soldati 2006).

The pathophysiology and histology of lung contusion is well described and occurs in various stages of development, with all phases initiated by parenchyma alveolar laceration and rupture. These pathological stages include (a) the trauma itself, which causes a hemorrhagic lacerated core by direct energy transfer to lung parenchyma; (b) an edematous phase with ensuing progressive infiltrate of the interstitium within one to two hours after the primary injury; (c) a flooding of the airspaces with blood, inflammatory cells, and tissue debris with maximal consolidation twenty-four to forty-eight hours after the lung injury (Soldati 2006). In addition, the extent and severity of lung damage and subsequent respiratory physiological abnormalities characteristically worsens in severity over the first seventy-two hours but then almost totally resolves by seven days, unless an additional concomitant disease process such as acute lung infection become superimposed (Cohn 1997). Within twenty-four hours, the pulmonary contusion score increases in severity in approximately 50 percent of patients (Tyburski 1999). Of 103 patients having pulmonary contusion on the twenty-four-hour chest x-ray, 11 did not have visible abnormalities on presentation to ED (Tyburski 1999). The chest CT scan is clearly superior to standard CXR in identifying pulmonary contusion (Cohn 1997). Frequently lung contusion will be missed on standard CXR with a frequency of 10.7 percent, thus relying upon chest CT as a more sensitive diagnostic modality (Tyburski 1999).

Abnormal Gas Exchange in Pulmonary Contusion: However, there exists little data categorically describing mechanisms of gas exchange abnormalities in lung contusion and the resultant mechanical defect of hypocompliant stiff lungs. In addition, few detailed studies have categorically characterized or validated the most effective modalities of invasive mechanical ventilator support, excluding when progression results in ARDS physiology and standard implementation of the lung protective ventilator strategy (Sharma 1996; ARDSnet 2000). Dependent upon maximal degree of lung injury, PaO_2/FiO_2 ratios are significantly and at times severely reduced (108 +/− 34.5 [Hernandez 2010] and 281 +/− 80 [Leone 2003]).

In an experimental animal model of blunt chest trauma and lung contusion, increases in both venous admixture ($\dot{Q}s/\dot{Q}t$) and absolute intrapulmonary shunt fractions were evident but of only modest degree, given very focal areas and limited volume of lung injury (Oppenheimer 1979). Blunt chest trauma damages pulmonary vasculature, causing the leakage of whole blood and plasma constituents into the adjacent interstitium and alveolar spaces. The consequent alveolar flooding is associated with reduced perfusion of the flooded region but little true shunt. Airspaces adjacent to the flooded regions have normal perfusion per unit volume but are less compliant, hence poorly ventilated. As a result, mean V/Q is reduced, and venous admixture is increased, causing arterial hypoxemia that responds easily to increased inspired oxygen administration (Oppenheimer 1979). However, in a clinical study of patients with varying degrees of pulmonary contusion, the actual degree of intrapulmonary shunt fraction is extremely variable with range of a low of 12 percent to a high of 41 percent in one select study (Wagner 1991), which authors related to interpatient variability in localized hypoxic pulmonary vasoconstriction (Wagner 1991). Yet, in a small subset of these patients, mechanisms of hypoxemia were demonstrated to result from increased venous to arterial shunting with measured values of Q̇s/Q̇t (venous admixture) between 17 and 20 percent (Garzon 1968).

Abnormal Respiratory Mechanics in Pulmonary Contusion: One study of twelve patients with "crushed-chest injuries" utilized ventilator-derived physiological variables to characterize lung mechanics in this population of patients (Garzon 1968). This study (Table 17.1) demonstrated significant decrease in lung compliance (Clung) and less dramatic but still significant increase in airway resistance (Raw) in these patients (on days two to four, lung compliance was reduced to values 0.06 +/- 0.03 L/cmH$_2$O versus control values 0.13 +/- 0.03 for women and 0.22 +/- 0.05 L/cmH$_2$O for men, and Raw 8.3 +/- 6.0 cmH$_2$O/L/sec compared to control values 3.2 +/- 0.4 for women and 1.9 +/- 0.6 for men [Garzon 1968]). In addition, significant reductions in PaO$_2$ were also demonstrated when obtained on room air with values for day one, day three, and day five measuring 56+/- 13 mmHg, 65+/- 14 mmHg, and 66 +/- 14 mmHg, respectively, which then normalized to 82 +/- 13 mmHg after two weeks. The decreased lung compliance was theorized to be directly resultant from lung injury and the increased Raw secondary to blood and retained secretions within the airways.

Table 17.1: Pulmonary Physiological Measurements in Patients with Lung Contusion (Garzon 1968)

	Clung (mL/cmH$_2$O)	Raw (cmH$_2$O/L/sec)
Controls	220 +/- 50 (males)	1.9 +/- 0.6 (males)
	130 +/- 30 (females)	3.2 +/- 0.4 (females)
Contusion	60 +/- 30	8.3 +/- 6.0

Flail Chest

Flail chest is produced by double fractures of three or more contiguous ribs or combined sternal and rib fractures. When several contiguous ribs are broken in multiple sites or detached from the sternum, a flail chest is created that does not move synchronously with the remainder of the thorax and often results in the detached, or flail, segment being pulled inward and paradoxical inward displacement during spontaneous inspiration. In the presence of paradoxical inward displacement of parts of the rib cage, the inspiratory muscles must shorten to a greater extent to achieve the same volume expansion (Tzelepis 1989; Cappello 1996). This implies greater velocity of shortening, greater work rate, and greater incremental respiratory muscle oxygen consumption (Tzelepis 1989). In an analysis of 427 patients hospitalized with blunt chest trauma from multiple etiologies, 95 of the 427 (22%) manifested flail chest (45 right sided, 31 left sided, 19 bilaterally); 86 percent of these 95 patients with flail chest also had evidence of significant pulmonary contusion by standard chest x-ray (Richardson 1982). However, both hypoxemia and respiratory insufficiency associated with flail chest is generally not directly resultant of the abnormal chest-wall mechanics but rather as a consequence and extent of the underlying pulmonary contusion (Bastos 2008; Donath 2009).

References

Bastos, R., J. H. Calhoon, and C. E. Baisden. 2008. "Flail Chest and Pulmonary Contusion." *Thoracic and Cardiovascular Surgery* 20: 39–45.

Cappello, M., and A. De Troyer. 1996. "Respiratory Muscle Response to Flail Chest." *American Journal of Respiratory and Critical Care Medicine* 153: 1897–1901.

Cohn, S. 1997. "Pulmonary Contusion: Review of the Clinical Entity." *Journal of Trauma* 42 (5): 973–979.

Donath, J., and A. Miller. 2009. "Restrictive Chest Wall Disorders." *Seminars in Respiratory and Critical Care Medicine* 30 (3): 275–292.

Garzon, A. A., B. Seltzer, and K. E. Karlson. 1968. "Physiopathology of Crushed Chest Injuries." *Annals of Surgery* 168 (1): 128–136.

Pape, H-C., D. Remmers, J. Rice, M. Ebisch, C. Krettek, and H. Tscherne. 2000. "Appraisal of Early Evaluation of Blunt Chest Trauma: Development of a Standardized Scoring System for Initial Clinical Decision Making." *Journal of Trauma* 49: 496–504.

Hernandez, G., R. Fernandez, P. Lopez-Reina, R. Cuena, A. Pedrosa, R. Ortiz, P. and Hiradier. 2010. "Noninvasive Ventilation Reduces Intubation in Chest Trauma-Related Hypoxemia." *Chest* 137 (1): 74–80.

Johnson, J. A., T. H. Cogbill, and E. R. Winga. 1986. "Determinants of Outcome after Pulmonary Contusion." *Journal of Trauma* 26 (8): 695–697.

Leone, M., J. Albanese, S. Rousseau, F. Antonini, M. Dubuc, B. Alliez, and C. Martin. 2003. "Pulmonary Contusion in Severe Head Trauma Patients." *Chest* 124: 2261–2266.

Miller, P. R., M. A. Croce, T. K. Bee, W. G. Qaisi, C. P. Smith, G. L. Collins, and T. C. Fabian. 2001. "ARDS after Pulmonary Contusion." *Journal of Trauma* 51: 223–230.

Oppenheimer, L., K. D. Craven, L. Forkert, and L. D. H. Wood. 1979. "Pathophysiology of Pulmonary Contusion in Dogs." *Journal of Applied Physiology: Respiratory Environmental and Exercise Physiology* 47 (4): 718–728.

Pepe, P. E., R. T. Potkin, D. H. Reus, L. D. Hudson, and C. J. Carrico. 1982. "Clinical Predictors of the Adult Respiratory Distress Syndrome." *American Journal of Surgery* 144: 124–130.

Richardson, J. D., L. Adams, and L. M. Flint. 1982. "Selective Management of Flail Chest and Pulmonary Contusion." *Annals of Surgery* 196 (4): 481–486.

Sharma, S., R. J. Mullins, and D. D. Trunkey. 1996. "Ventilatory Management of Pulmonary Contusion Patients." *American Journal of Surgery* 172: 529–532.

Soldati, G., A. Testa, F. R. Silva, L. Carbone, G. Portale, N. G. Silveri. 2006. "Chest Ultrasonography in Lung Contusion." *Chest* 130: 533–538.

The Acute Respiratory Distress Syndrome Network. 2000. "Ventilation with Lower Tidal Volumes as Compared with Traditional Tidal Volumes for Acute Lung Injury and the Acute Respiratory Distress Syndrome." *New England Journal of Medicine* 342: 1301–1308.

Tyburski, J. G., J. Collinge, R. F. Wilson, S. Eachempati. 1999. "Pulmonary Contusion: Quantifying the Lesions on Chest X-Ray Films and the Factors Affecting Prognosis." *Journal of Trauma* 46 (5): 833–838.

Tzelepis, G. E., J. Collinge, R. F. Wilson, S. Eachempati. 1989. "Chest Wall Distortion in Patients with Flail Chest." *American Review of Respiratory Disease* 140: 31–37.

Wagner, R. B., B. Slivko, P. M. Jamieson. M. S. Dills, F. H. Edwards. 1991. "Effect of Lung Contusion on Pulmonary Hemodynamics." *Annals of Thoracic Surgery* 52: 51–58.

CHAPTER 18

Extreme/Morbid Obesity

• • •

As READILY PORTRAYED IN BOTH public/lay press and medical literature, the incidence of obesity of all degrees and severity and across all ages in the United States and probably worldwide in industrialized countries is increasing epidemically. In an epidemiological report for 2009–2010, 16.9 percent of children and adolescents between the ages of two and nineteen were defined as obese (Ogden 2012) and 35.5 percent of adult men and 35.8 percent of adult women were considered obese (Flegal 2012). It only stands to reason that more and more patients with obesity will come under the care of critical-care physicians and intensivists. Publications have already documented that up to 25 percent of all ICU admissions are obese (Marik 1998; Goulenok 2004; Ray 2005; Martino 2011), and between 4 and 13 percent are described as severely obese (El-Solh 2001; Ray 2005; Martino 2011). This also includes patients with extreme obesity. Perhaps surprisingly, obesity per se in some publications does not always portend an increased ICU mortality (Amundson 2010). However, what is very clear is that obesity does indeed have significant repercussions and negative effects upon multiple aspects of pulmonary physiology, including mechanics and gas exchange (Ashburn 2010). In addition, it must be realized that any demonstrated mechanical or gas-exchange abnormalities in the awake, upright, or sitting extremely obese patient will only become markedly exaggerated and worsened in the supine, sedated critical-care arena (Ashburn 2010). Thus, even in the absence of intrinsic lung disease, extremely obese patients would appear to represent a group of ICU patients at high risk for pulmonary complications (Pelosi 1996; Lee 2008). A marked reduction in expiratory reserve volume (ERV) is the most consistently demonstrated static pulmonary function tests (PFTs) abnormality of extremely obese patients which values less than 400 mL closely correlating with magnitude of hypoxemia rather than BMI per se (Holley 1967; Zerah 1993; Pelosi 1996; Koening 2001; Jones 2006).

In relation to measurements of total respiratory systems compliance (Ctotal, rs), virtually all studies have shown significant reductions in comparison to nonobese controls with the bulk of this reduction attributed surprisingly to reduced lung compliance (Clung) and not necessarily reduced chest-wall compliance (Ccw) as the predominate physiological abnormality. Again, note that in one study there was no observed differences in Ccw between normal volunteers and extremely obese subjects and also that Ccw did not correlate with BMI, thus raising speculation about different obesity phenotypes, which are known to exist between extreme obesity with or without obesity hypoventilation syndrome (OHS) (Suratt 1984).

In a study of stable, nonacutely ill subjects still considered definitive and classic as defining pulmonary physiological derangements in obese patients, (a) normal-weighted subjects were compared to (b) obese subjects without OHS and (c) obese subjects with OHS (Sharp 1964, Figure 3). As frequently reported, measurements of static lung volumes demonstrated that ERV was proportionately reduced between these three groups: (a) 1.72 L versus (b) 0.75 L versus (c) 0.51 L. With the thorax defined as applying to all structures surrounding the lung, including rib cage, diaphragm, and abdominal contents, significant abnormalities were reported as recorded in the accompanying Table 18.1. In addition, given the markedly abnormal lung mechanics, significant increases in work of breathing (WOB), whether partitioned into lung-related WOB or total thoracic respiratory WOB, were observed for obese patients in comparison to healthy control individuals (Sharp 1964).

Table 18.1: Pulmonary Physiology Measurements in Patients with Obesity +/− Obesity Hypoventilation Syndrome (OHS) Compared to Healthy Volunteers (Sharp 1964)

	Healthy	Obese (−) OHS	Obese (+) OHS
Ctotal (L/cmH$_2$O)	0.104 +/− 0.005	0.081 +/− 0.007	0.045 +/− 0.002
	(0.080–0.156)	(0.059–0.130)	(0.038–0.051)
Clung (L/cmH$_2$O)	0.211 +/− 0.02	0.157 +/− 0.02	0.122 +/− 0.036
	(0.125–0.310)	(0.107–0.250)	(0.097–0.142)
Ccw (L/cmH$_2$O)	0.214 +/− 0.014	0.196 +/− 0.018	0.075 +/− 0.010
	(0.140–0.270)	(0.140–0.274)	(0.052–0.108)
Raw (cmH$_2$O/L/sec)	1.3 +/− 0.1	3.8 +/− 0.3	3.8 +/− 0.5
WOB (lung) (kg-m/L at 20 BPM)	0.035 +/− 0.003	0.054 +/− 0.006	0.085 +/− 0.010
WOB (thoracic-cw) (kg-m/L at 20 BPM)	0.038 +/− 0.004	0.043 +/− 0.006	0.127 +/− 0.22
WOB (total) (kg-m/L at 20 BPM)	0.073 +/− 0.005	0.095 +/− 0.010	0.212 +/− 0.021

In general, in obese OHS patients, the elastance workload of the lung was doubled (50% compliance of normal) compared to normal and the thorax / chest wall three times (35% compliance of normal) the healthy subject values.

In a corroborative study, similar values again demonstrating significant reductions in total, lung, and chest-wall compliance and correlative increases in WOB were also observed again in a select group of obese, awake volunteers compared to nonobese control subjects. As expected, the combined mechanical workload placed upon the respiratory muscles was also increased, normal, healthy subjects = 0.227 kg-m/L versus obese patients = 0.540 kg-m/L (Naimark 1960).

Table 18.2: Pulmonary Physiology Measurements in Obese Patients Compared to Healthy Volunteers (Naimark 1960)

	Healthy	Obese
C_{total} (L/cmH$_2$O)	0.119 +/− 0.045 (0.065–0.228)	0.052 +/− 0.025 (0.021–0.107)
C_{lung} (L/cmH$_2$O)	0.283 +/− 0.088 (0.140–0.441)	0.200 +/− 0.113 (0.084–0.367)
C_{cw} (L/cmH$_2$O)	0.240 +/− 0.110 (0.140–0.550)	0.077 +/− 0.041 (0.024–0.151)
WOB (total) (kg-m/L)	0.227	0.540

Surprisingly, the mechanical thoracic abnormalities in obese patients are not simply related to reduced compliance; studies have also consistently demonstrated increases in airway resistance as additional factors and workloads eventually contributing to exercise limitation and possible hypercapnia. This increase in Raw (56% higher than controls) was also shown to be directly related to decrease in ERV given the concomitant reduction in overall lung volume and the importance of Raw dependent upon lung size/volume (Zerah 1993). This physiological abnormality was thought to be directly resultant from premature airway closure of peripheral airways in these gravity-dependent basilar lung units (Zerah 1993).

In postoperative obese patients receiving invasive mechanical ventilation, the total resistance of entire respiratory system (Rmaxrs) was significantly higher in obese patients, measuring 4.4 +/− 0.9 versus 1.6 +/− 3.7 cmH_2O/L/sec with reciprocal expected increases in lung-specific Raw also being threefold higher in obese versus nonobese patients, measuring 9.6 +/− 4.1 versus 3.2 +/− 0.9 cmH_2O/L/sec (Pelosi 1996).

In addition, this premature peripheral airway collapse also created units of nonventilated alveoli but preserved blood flow, especially in relation to gravitational factors that create both increased intrapulmonary true shunt and increased venous admixture ($Q\dot{s}/Q\dot{t}$) that represent continued blood flow to areas of significantly reduced V/Q, again creating shuntlike physiology and resultant hypoxemia (Barrera 1973; Koening 2001; Ashburn 2010). Calculated measurements for these various contributing components to hypoxemia in extremely obese patients demonstrated increased measurements of true intrapulmonary shunt from normal values of 2.3 percent to 11.5 percent in severely obese patients and increases in venous admixture, reflecting continued perfusion to lung units with low V/Q from 6.6 percent to 30.4 percent in obesity (Barrera 1973).

In the same study evaluating respiratory mechanics in postoperative obese patients receiving invasive ventilation, reduced total respiratory system compliance was again demonstrated, being contributed to jointly by reduced lung compliance and reduced thoracic-wall compliance consisting of chest wall, ribs, diaphragm, and abdominal contents. However, again, the lung component was predominant with extremely obese patients, with FRC also markedly lower than nonobese patients (0.665 +/− 0.191 L vs 1.691 +/− 0.325 L) (Pelosi 1996). Static compliance of the respiratory system was reduced approximately 50 percent compared to nonobese 34.5 +/− 5.1 mL/cmH_2O versus 66.4 +/− 14.4 mL/cmH_2O (Pelosi 1996). This reduction in total compliance of the entire respiratory system was decreased mostly because of a decrease in static lung compliance with Cst, lung values 55.3 +/− 15.3 mL/cmH$_2$0 versus 106.6 +/− 31.7 mL/cmH$_2$O (Pelosi 1996) but also contributed to by reduced chest-wall compliance Cst, cw 112.4 +/− 47.4 versus 190.7 +/− 45.1 mL/cmH$_2$O (Pelosi 1996, Figure 2).

Table 18.3: Pulmonary Physiology Measurements in Postoperative Obese and Nonobese Patients (Pelosi 1996)

	Post-Op: Nonobese	Post-Op: Obese
Ctotal (L/cmH$_2$O)	0.0664 +/− 0.0144	0.0345 +/− 0.0051
Clung (L/cmH$_2$O)	0.106 +/− 0.0317	0.0553 +/− 0.0153
Ccw (L/cmH$_2$O)	0.1907 +/− 0.0451	0.1124 +/− 0.0474
WOB (Total)[J/L]	0.52 +/− 0.1	1.30 +/− 0.19
WOB (lung)[J/L]	0.34 +/− 0.08	0.90 +/− 0.25
WOB (cw)[J/L]	0.18 +/− 0.04	0.39 +/− 0.13

However, interestingly, the relative percent contributions of both Cst, lung and Cst, cw were similar between obese and nonobese patients: obese Clung = 65 percent, Ccw = 35 percent; and nonobese controls Clung = 64 percent, Ccw = 36 percent (Pelosi 1996). The proposed mechanism for the universal finding of reduced lung compliance is attributable to premature airway closure in the bases or gravity-dependent portions of the lung, which shifts the pressure-volume (P-V) curve to a less steep / more disadvantageous position and thus requires greater pressure gradients to expand. When WOB was portioned into various relative components, 55 percent was attributed to decreased lung compliance, 30 percent attributed to decreased chest-wall compliance, and 15 percent attributed to increased respiratory airway resistance (Pelosi 1996).

Similar results of reduced total respiratory system compliance (Crs, tot) and increases in both total WOB and oxygen cost of breathing were reported in additional studies (Table 18.4), which again demonstrated the marked increase in respiratory work and respiratory muscle energy expenditure in obese subjects.

Table 18.4. Measurements of Respiratory Mechanics and Respiratory Muscle Energy Expenditure in both Healthy Subjects and Patients without (−) obesity hypoventilation syndrome (OHS) or with (+) OHS (Koening 2001)

	Healthy	Obese (−OHS)	Obese (+OHS)
Crs, tot (L/cmH$_2$O)	0.11	0.05	0.06
WOBtotal (J/L)	0.43	0.74	1.64
O$_2$ Cost Breathing (mLO$_2$/L)	1.1	4.5	10.4

Another method to measure the oxygen cost of breathing is to obtain a basal resting level of total body oxygen consumption ($\dot{V}O_2$) and then obtain the same measurements when patients are intubated and sedated. Using this method and subtracting both values should give an overall estimation of the specific component of $\dot{V}O_2$ relegated to breathing. Using such an approach, extreme-obesity patients demonstrated higher measurements of oxygen cost of breathing than normal, healthy individuals with $\dot{V}O_2$ measuring 354.6 mLO$_2$/min versus 221.5 mLO$_2$/min, but more specifically, upon assuming controlled ventilation, the $\dot{V}O_2$ for morbidly obese patients dropped significantly to 297.2 mLO$_2$/min, but healthy controls remained the same at 219.8 mLO$_2$/min (Kress 1999). These results are consistent with the relatively low $\dot{V}O_2$resp in healthy individuals and the increased metabolic load placed upon the respiratory muscles to expand the overall hypocompliant respiratory system of severely obese patients.

REFERENCES

Amundson, D. E., S. Djurkovic, and G. N. Matwiyoff. 2010. "The Obesity Paradox." *Critical Care Clinics* 26: 583–596.

Ashburn, D. D., A. DeAntonio, and M. J. Reed. 2010. "Pulmonary System and Obesity." *Critical Care Clinics* 26: 597–602.

Barrera, F., P. Hillyer, G. Ascanio, and J. Bechtel. 1973. "The Distribution of Ventilation, Diffusion, and Blood Flow in Obese Patients with Normal and Abnormal Blood Gases." *American Review of Respiratory Disease* 108: 819–830.

El-Solh, A., P. Sikka, E. Bozkanat, W. Jaafar, and J. Davies. 2001. "Morbid Obesity in the Medical ICU." *Chest* 120 (6): 1989–1997.

Flegal, K. M., M. D. Carroll, B. K. Kit, and C. L. Ogden. 2012. "Prevalence of Obesity and Trends in the Distribution of Body Mass Index among US Adults, 1999–2010." *Journal of the American Medical Association* 307 (5): 491–497.

Goulenok, C., M. Monchi, J-D. Chiche, J-P. Mira, J-F. Dhainaut, A. Cariou. 2004. "Influence of Overweight on ICU Mortality." *Chest* 125: 1441–1445.

Holley, H. S., J. Milic-Emili, M. R. Becklake, and D. V. Bates. 1967. "Regional Distribution of Pulmonary Ventilation and Perfusion in Obesity." *Journal of Clinical Investigation* 46 (4): 475–481.

Jones, R. L., and M. M. U. Nzekwu. 2006. "The Effects of Body Mass Index on Lung Volumes." *Chest* 130: 827–833.

Koening, S. M. 2001. "Pulmonary Complications of Obesity." *American Journal of Medical Science* 321 (4): 249–279.

Kress, J. P., A. S. Pohlman, J. Alverdy, J. B. Hall. 1999. "The Impact of Morbid Obesity on Oxygen Cost of Breathing at Rest." *American Journal of Respiratory and Critical Care Medicine* 160: 883–886.

Lee, W. Y., and B. Mokhlesi. 2008. "Diagnosis and Management of Obesity Hypoventilation Syndrome in the ICU." *Critical Care Clinics* 24: 533–549.

Marik, P., and J. Varon. 1998. "The Obese Patient in the ICU." *Chest* 113: 492–498.

Martino, J. L., R. D. Stapleton, M. Wang, A. G. Day, N. E. Cahill, A. E. Dixon, B. T. Suratt, and D. K. Heyland. 2011. "Extreme Obesity and Outcomes in Critically Ill Patients." *Chest* 140 (5): 1198–1206.

Naimark, A., and R. M. Cherniack. 1960. "Compliance of the Respiratory System and its Components in Health and Obesity." *Journal of Applied Physiology* 15: 377–382.

Ogden, C. L., M. D. Carroll, B. K. Kit, K. M. Flegal. 2012. "Prevalence of Obesity and Trends in Body Mass Index among US Children and Adolescents, 1999–2010." *Journal of the American Medical Association* 307 (5): 483–490.

Pelosi, P., M. Croci, I. Ravagnan, P. Vicardi, L. Gattinoni. 1996. "Total Respiratory System, Lung, and Chest Wall Mechanics in Sedated-Paralyzed Postoperative Morbidly Obese Patients." *Chest* 109: 144–151.

Ray, D. E., S. C. Matchett, K. Baker, T. Wasser, and M. J. Young. 2005. "The Effect of Body Mass Index on Patient Outcomes in a Medical ICU." *Chest* 127: 2125–2131.

Sharp, J. T., J. P. Henry, S. K. Sweany, W. R. Meadows, and R. J. Pietras. 1964. "The Total Work of Breathing in Normal and Obese Men." *Journal of Clinical Investigation* 43 (4): 728–739.

Suratt, P. M., S. C. Wilhoit, H. S. Hsiao, R. L. Atkinson, and D. F. Rochester. 1984. "Compliance of Chest Wall in Obese Subjects." *Journal of Applied Physiology* 57 (2): 403–407.

Zerah, F., A. Harf, L. Perlemuter, H. Lorino, A. M. Lorino, and G. Atlan. 1993. "Effects of Obesity on Respiratory Resistance." *Chest* 103: 1470–1476.

CHAPTER 19

Cystic Fibrosis

• • •

CYSTIC FIBROSIS (CF) RESULTS FROM an inherited disease-causing mutation in the gene coding for the CF transmembrane conductance regulatory protein (CFTR). CF is an inherited monogenetic homozygous recessive multisystem disease affecting all the exocrine organs, including sweat glands, the biliary system, the pancreas, the intestines, reproductive systems, and the entirety of the respiratory system (nose, sinus, and airways of the lung) (O'Sullivan 2009). CF affects approximately thirty thousand individual patients in the United States and sixty thousand worldwide. Despite significant advances in therapies and lung transplantation, CF remains a life-limiting disease with median survival of 39.3 years but, importantly, a median age of death of 29.1 years (CFF Patient Registry 2014). Respiratory failure and complications of lung transplantation remain the most common cause of death in patients with CF, approximately 70 percent and 12 percent, respectively. Each year approximately two hundred patients with CF undergo bilateral lung transplantation, and, given the opportunity for this therapy, many CF patients are being admitted to intensive-care units (ICUs), often receiving invasive mechanical ventilation and extracorporeal membrane oxygenation (ECMO) as a "bridge" to transplantation. In addition, an increasing number of CF patients with severe lung disease are being managed in critical-care settings for complications of acute infectious exacerbations (AECF) of their existent chronic suppurative CF-related bronchiectasis. The institution of invasive mechanical ventilation as life-sustaining support for CF patients is associated with high mortality, but there is a high probability that it will still be offered to many such patients (Berlinski 2002; Texereau 2006; Efrati 2010; Sheikh 2011).

To date there exist few objective, evidence-based recommendations in relation to the respiratory management and care of these critically ill patients presenting not only with respiratory failure but other major complications also such as malnutrition, depression, and CF-related diabetes (CFRD) (Sood 2001; Kremer 2008). Yet few studies have intensively investigated the mechanisms of abnormalities in either gas exchange or pulmonary mechanics in critically ill, mechanically ventilated CF patients. With this as background, focus will be extended to an understanding of both gas exchange and lung mechanical abnormalities in adult patients with severe CF lung disease (usually defined as percent predicted $FEV1 < 40\%$), acknowledging the inability to make direct concrete analogies between these outpatient studies and CF patients directly receiving ICU care.

The hallmark pathological lesion of CF lung disease is the abnormal permanent enlargement/dilatation of the small (bronchiolectasis) and large (bronchiectasis) airways associated with irreversible/fixed structural damage/destruction resultant from sustained airway infection, inflammation, and suppuration (Gibson 2003). Similar to patients with acute exacerbations of COPD, patients with CF lung disease frequently develop, acutely or subacutely, (a) worsening subjective symptoms such as cough, sputum, fatigue, or dyspnea; (b) new objective physical signs such as fever, weight loss, tachypnea, tachycardia, or new findings on lung auscultation; (c) changes in laboratory or radiographic assessment such as leukocytosis, hypoxemia, or increased infiltrates on chest x-ray; or (d) most importantly, worsening lung physiology based upon formal pulmonary function test (PFT) measurements. Although lacking a rigid definition for an acute infectious exacerbation of known CF-related bronchiectasis (AECF), some combination of these findings supports a diagnosis of AECF, frequently requiring inpatient hospitalization and the acute initiation of intravenous antibiotics. Depending upon the severity of these symptoms, signs, and findings, patients with CF often require ICU-level care and also commonly the necessity for invasive mechanical ventilatory support. Of note, in patients with AECF, the level of inflammation and magnitude of bacterial burden far exceed that of any other pulmonary disease.

Abnormal Gas Exchange in Cystic Fibrosis

Most studies investigating mechanisms of hypoxemia in patients with CF have utilized the multiple inert gas elimination technique (MIGET). Early studies recruiting only small numbers of CF patients with a wide range of pulmonary disease severity (based upon percent predicted FEV1) have seemed to suggest that that intrapulmonary shunt was the predominant cause of hypoxemia with a small variable contribution by low V/Q lung units (Dantzker 1982). However, more recent investigations using larger numbers of patients with higher levels of lung disease severity (percent predicted FEV1 < 50%) have refuted this initial observation and have established that the primary mechanism of hypoxemia in both chronically stable patients and patients with AECF is V/Q inequality without any evidence of diffusion impairment (Lagerstrand 1999; Soni 2008). In the first-referenced study of ten CF patients older than sixteen years with demonstrated hypoxemia (mean PaO_2 = 76.5 +/- 7.5 mmHg), intrapulmonary shunt measured only 1.4 +/- 0.4 percent of the total cardiac output (Lagerstrand 1999). In the latter-referenced study involving fifteen adult CF subjects (mean PaO_2 = 69.5 +/- 9.6 mmHg), intrapulmonary shunt was negligible with mean values = 0.5 +/- 0.7 percent of the total cardiac output, with six subjects demonstrating no shunt whatsoever (Soni 2008).

Similar to all critically ill ICU patients, there exist multiple factors, often combined, contributing to the development of hypercapnia in CF patients. Although not directly measured, but purely from extrapolation using a prediction equation to estimate dead space fraction (Vd/Vt) in ICU patients, there is a suggestion that marked increases in Vd/Vt contribute to the generation of hypercapnia in mechanically ventilated patients. This same study suggests that serial measurements of Vd/Vt can also provide prognostic information in relation to mortality (Vender 2014). In one study of sixteen stable and not acutely ill CF patients between the ages of fifteen and thirty-five years without hypercapnia ($PaCO_2$ = 42 +/− 6 and 41 +/− 5 mmHg) but with severe CF lung disease (FEV1 = 28 +/− 7% predicted and 41 +/− 12% predicted), measurements of dead-space fraction were not significantly elevated, with recorded values of 0.32 +/− 0.05 and 0.27 +/− 0.05; these values of Vd/Vt did not correlate with resting values of static pulmonary function testing measures (Coates 1988). These studies highlight the limited information conclusively documenting the specific gas exchange abnormalities in ICU-level critically ill CF patients requiring invasive mechanical ventilation.

Abnormal Respiratory Mechanics in Cystic Fibrosis

Given the genetically mediated biochemical abnormalities associated with CF and the high levels of catabolism and increased metabolic activity generated from the marked levels of heightened lung infection and inflammation, most studies have measured increased levels of resting energy expenditures in patients with CF compared to healthy control subjects. In specific relation to the energy expenditures in CF patients for the work of breathing (WOB) and the oxygen cost of breathing resultant from these abnormalities in lung mechanics, studies have demonstrated that as lung function declines (as assessed by measurements of FEV1), there is an increase in the respiratory muscle load (both WOBelastic and WOBtotal). In a group of thirty-two CF subjects with percent predicted FEV1 = 28.7 +/− 10.2 (range 12–49), this increase was predominately contributed to by decreases in dynamic lung compliance (Cldyn) (Hart 2002). In this study, WOB total = 12.6 +/− 5.0 J/min (range 4.3–21.7); WOBelastic = 7.6 +/− 3.0 J/min (range 2.8–13.8); and WOBresistance = 5.1 +/− 2.5 J/min (range 0.8–10.7). A correlative study with data reproduced in Table 19.1 also reported increased measured values for oxygen cost of breathing for ten CF patients with moderate-to-severe lung disease severity (percent predicted FEV1 = 40.0 +/− 18.1) when compared to healthy control subjects.

Table 19.1. Oxygen Cost of Breathing in Adult CF Patients Compared to Healthy Subjects (Bell 1996)

	Oxygen Cost of Breathing	
	mL O_2/L	mL O_2/minute
Healthy Subjects	2.1 +/− 0.7	14.0 +/− 3.6
CF Patients	2.9 +/− 1.4	28.5 +/− 11.7

REFERENCES

Bell, S. C., M. J. Saunders, J. S. Elborn, and D. J. Shale. 1996. "Resting Energy Expenditure and Oxygen Cost of Breathing in Patients with Cystic Fibrosis." *Thorax* 51: 126–131.

Berlinski, A., L. L. Fan, C. A. Kozinetz, and C. M. Oermann. 2002. "Invasive Mechanical Ventilation for Acute Respiratory Failure in Children with Cystic Fibrosis: Outcome Analysis and Case-Control Study." *Pediatric Pulmonology* 34: 297–303.

Coates, A. L., G. Canny, R. Zinman, R. Grisdale, K. Desmond, D. Roumeliotis, and H. Levison. 1988. "The Effects of Chronic Airflow Limitation, Increased Dead Space, and the Pattern of Ventilation on Gas Exchange During Maximal Exercise in Advanced Cystic Fibrosis." *American Review of Respiratory Disease* 138: 1524–1531.

Cystic Fibrosis Foundation (CF) Patient Registry. 2014. Cystic Fibrosis Foundation, Bethesda, MD.

Dantzker, D. R., G. A. Patten, and J. S. Bower. 1982. "Gas Exchange at Rest and During Exercise in Adults with Cystic Fibrosis." *American Review of Respiratory Disease* 125: 400–405.

Efrati, O., I. Bylin, E. Segal, D. Vilozni, D. Modan-Moses, A. Vardi, A. Szeinberg, and G. Paret. 2010. "Outcome of Patients with Cystic Fibrosis Admitted to the Intensive Care Unit: Is Invasive Mechanical Ventilation a Risk Factor for Death in Patients Waiting Lung Transplantation?" *Heart and Lung* 39: 153–159.

Hart, N., M. I. Polkey, A. Clement, M. Boule, J. Moxham, F. Lofaso, and B. Fauroux. 2002. "Changes in Pulmonary Mechanics with Increasing Disease Severity in Children and Young Adults with Cystic Fibrosis." *American Journal of Respiratory and Critical Care Medicine* 166: 61–66.

Gibson, R. L., J. L. Burns, and B. W. Ramsey. 2003. "Pathophysiology and Management of Pulmonary Infections in Cystic Fibrosis." *American Journal of Respiratory and Critical Care Medicine* 168: 918–951.

Kremer, T. M., R. G. Zwerdling, P. H. Michelson, and B. P. O'Sullivan. 2008. "Intensive Care Management of the Patient with Cystic Fibrosis." *Journal of Intensive Care Medicine* 23: 159–177.

Lagerstrand, L., L. Hjelte, and H. Jorulf. 1999. "Pulmonary Gas Exchange in Cystic Fibrosis: Basal Status and the Effect of I. V. Antibiotics and Inhaled Amiloride." *European Respiratory Journal.* 14: 686–692.

O'Sullivan, B. P., and S. D. Freedman. 2009. "Cystic Fibrosis." *Lancet* 373: 1891–1904.

Sheikh, H. S., N. D. Tiangco, C. Harrell, and R. L. Vender. 2011. "Severe Hypercapnia in Critically Ill Adult Cystic Fibrosis Patients." *Journal of Clinical Medical Research*, June 6. doi: 10.4021/jocm612w.

Soni, R., C. J. Dobbib, M. A. Milross, I. H. Young, and P. P. T. Bye. 2008. "Gas Exchange in Stable Patients with Moderate-to-Severe Lung Disease from Cystic Fibrosis." *Journal of Cystic Fibrosis* 7: 285–291.

Sood, N, L. J. Paradowski, J. R. Yankaskas. 2001. "Outcome of Intensive Care Unit Care in Adults with Cystic Fibrosis Admitted to the Intensive Care Unit." *American Journal of Respiratory and Critical Care Medicine* 163: 335–338.

Texereau, J., D. Jamal, G. Choukroun, P. R. Burgel, J. L. Diehl, A. Rabbat, P. Loirat, et al. 2006. "Determinants of Mortality for Adults with Cystic Fibrosis Admitted in Intensive Care Unit: A Multicenter Study." *Respiratory Research* 7: 14.

Vender, R. L., M. F. Betancourt, E. B. Lehman, C. Harrell, D. Galvan, and D. C. Frankenfield. 2014. "Prediction Equation to Estimate Dead Space to Tidal Volume Fraction Correlates with Mortality in Critically Ill Patients." *Journal of Critical Care* 29 (2): e1-317e3.

About the Author

• • •

ROBERT L. VENDER, MD, is an actively practicing board-certified pulmonary and critical care physician. While he has spent most of his career in academic medical centers, working in settings ranging from small rural institutions to large city hospitals has provided him with a broad focus.

With thirty years of experience behind him, he still maintains an enthusiasm and fascination for the science and practice of medicine and the uniqueness of each patient for whom he has the honor of providing care. In their service, he continues to expand his knowledge and abilities daily.

Respiratory Physiology for the Intensivist makes a valuable contribution to the practical understanding of care and management of critically ill patients in an ICU setting without going into specific clinical practice patterns or guidelines.

Made in the USA
Middletown, DE
30 May 2017